CONTENTS

PREFACE

Many books have been written about AIDS and the suffering of the people, families, communities, and countries affected by it. Today these issues remain as important as ever, but this book has rather a different theme. In *Virus Hunt* we go behind the scenes to reveal the work of the international teams of scientists that have painstakingly uncovered the origin of the viruses that cause AIDS.

The idea behind the book is to tell the story of scientific discoveries over several decades that have eventually revealed the true history of the AIDS pandemic. So this is not about what happened after the first cases were described in the early 1980s but rather about events that occurred around one hundred years earlier that silently laid the foundations for the massive pandemic we are experiencing today.

AIDS hit the headlines in 1981 when it was first recognized in the US. Very rapidly similar epidemics were reported in several other countries. Human immunodeficiency virus, or HIV, the causative virus, was discovered within two years, but its exact origins were hotly debated for the next thirty years.

Virus Hunt recounts the scientific trail that eventually solved the mystery of the origin of HIV. Cracking it required a wide range of experts from laboratory scientists to epidemiologists, animal ecologists, and evolutionary biologists, all working together as a team. The journey has been a long and complicated one, fraught with wrong turnings and false trails. At times progress was halted by lack of available tools and had to wait for further technological advances before it could take the next logical step. Along the way many previously unknown viruses have been discovered, not least twelve 'new' HIVs that are presently spreading among us.

As a virologist I watched from the sidelines as the HIV story unfolded and found it frankly riveting. As each new piece of the puzzle fell into place we got closer to finding out just when, where, how, and why HIV first infected us and then spread like wildfire, until a logical picture finally emerged. Only then did the history of HIV from the original infection of a single person to the present total of over 60 million infections make any kind of sense.

Virus Hunt takes us on a journey from the US where AIDS was first identified to Africa to uncover its origins. We then travel back in time, following HIV from its discovery in France to the rainforests of west central Africa to search for its closest living relatives. Finally, we follow its global journey from rural west central Africa to local urban centres, and then on to the Caribbean. From here it jumped to the US where the discovery of AIDS closes the circle.

I am not claiming that this story is now complete or that it will not change in the future, because there remain holes to be filled in, and, of course, further discoveries may alter our views. But still it is a wonderful story of scientific endeavour which in my opinion is well worth the telling.

'If a man will begin with certainties, he shall end in doubts, but if he will be content to begin with doubts he shall end in certainties' (Sir Frances Bacon, 1561–1626).

ACKNOWLEDGEMENTS

I would like to thank the following experts for their comments and advice on the manuscript of this book:

Cristian Apetrei, Tulane National Primate Research Center, USA; Kevin De Cock, Center for Global Health, Centers for Disease Control and Prevention, US; João Dinis de Sousa, Katholieke Universiteit Leuven, Belgium; Beatrice Hahn, University of Pennsylvania, US; John Iliffe, University of Cambridge, UK; Philippe Lemey, Katholieke Universiteit Leuven, Belgium; Martine Peeters, University of Montpellier, France; Peter Piot, London School of Hygiene and Tropical Medicine, UK; Andrew Rambaut, University of Edinburgh, UK; Marco Salemi, University of Florida, US; Robin Weiss, University College London, UK; Mike Worobey, University of Arizona, USA.

I am grateful for the constant support provided by Latha Menon and Emma Marchant at Oxford University Press and also thank the following for reading and commenting on the draft manuscript: William Alexander, Jeanne Bell, Richard Boyd, Rod Dalitz, Frances Fowler, Ingo Johannessen, Barbara Judge, Jane Mitchell, and J Alero Thomas.

I am particularly indebted to John Mokili, San Diego State University, California, USA, for organizing my fact-finding trip to the Democratic Republic of Congo and also to Paul Sharp, University of Edinburgh, whose fascinating research seminars first inspired me to write this book. Paul has also given generously of his time with support and advice during the writing of the book and has provided the evolutionary trees.

The research undertaken for this book was supported by a grant from the Wellcome Trust.

LIST OF FIGURES

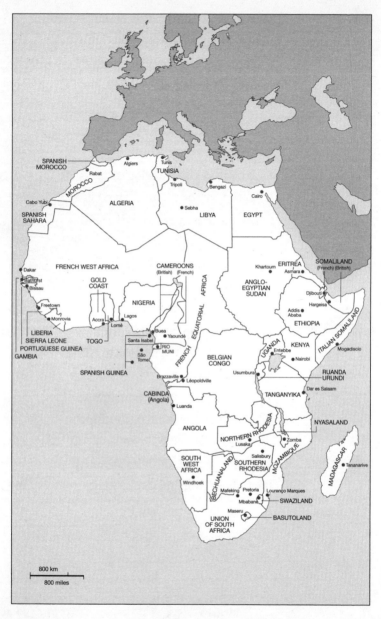

MAP 1 Map showing the countries of Africa in **1955**.
Courtesy of Library of Congress, Geography and map Division.

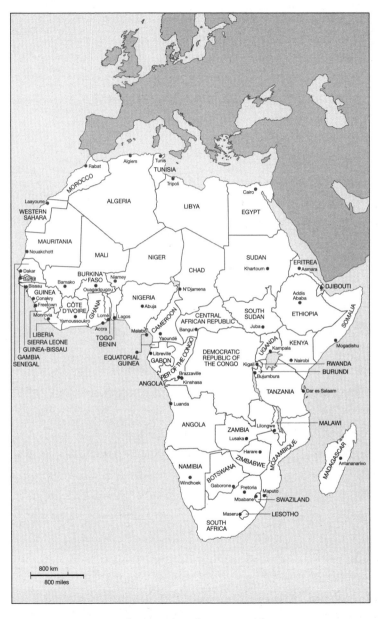

MAP 2 Map showing the of countries Africa in **2013**.
Courtesy of Central Intelligence Agency.

Introduction
A New Disease

It is now over thirty years since AIDS burst onto the scene completely unheralded. It soon dominated the headlines. In the Western world we were congratulating ourselves on getting to grips with infectious diseases one day, and the next a new, fatal infection appeared among us. Those of us working as infectious disease doctors will never forget the frenetic days in 1981 when our lack of knowledge left us feeling totally impotent. With the epidemic spreading, young men dying, the death toll rising, and new revelations emerging, all at breakneck speed, we had no idea where the disease came from, how it spread, or how to stop it. However, I am conscious that anyone presently under the age of 40 years did not experience this drama first hand, and so this introduction provides a short summary of events as they unfolded in the West, and gives a feel for the panic and finger-pointing that followed.

Early in 1981 doctors in Los Angeles, US, reported a completely new disease—an immune deficiency so severe that its victims died rapidly from overwhelming infections. No sooner had the

LA group's report appeared than similar reports came from San Francisco and New York. Rare infections like *Pneumocystis* pneumonia and an unusually aggressive tumour called Kaposi's sarcoma topped the growing list of diseases that proved fatal in these patients as their immune systems collapsed completely. When doctors in London and several other European capitals also reported cases it was clear that a new, inexplicable epidemic had been unleashed.

Uniquely, the disease specifically targeted sexually active gay men and although it was officially named AIDS (acquired immunodeficiency syndrome), in 1982 the label 'gay plague' was soon coined by the press. No one had a clue why the disease was restricted to gay men but it was soon apparent that sufferers 'lived life in the fast lane', regularly visiting bath houses and sex clubs and having multiple sexual partners. Some claimed a lifetime count of well over a thousand different partners. So how was AIDS related to this fast-lane lifestyle? Was it caused by 'poppers', the drugs that gay men often used to heighten sexual pleasure, or was there a 'new' sexually transmitted microbe on the loose?

Among the first men diagnosed with AIDS was 'patient zero', a gay Canadian airline steward who reckoned to have had around 2,500 sexual encounters in his 10 years of gay sex. He developed enlarged lymph glands in 1979, Kaposi's sarcoma in 1980, and died of AIDS in 1984. Researchers retracing his travels found he had had sex with at least forty of the earliest AIDS cases in ten cities across two continents, strongly suggesting that he was spreading a sexually transmitted infectious agent[1] (Figure 1).

When AIDS was first recognized in 1981, the risk of catching it seemed to be restricted to gay men, but very quickly it became a whole lot scarier. Within six months injecting drug users joined

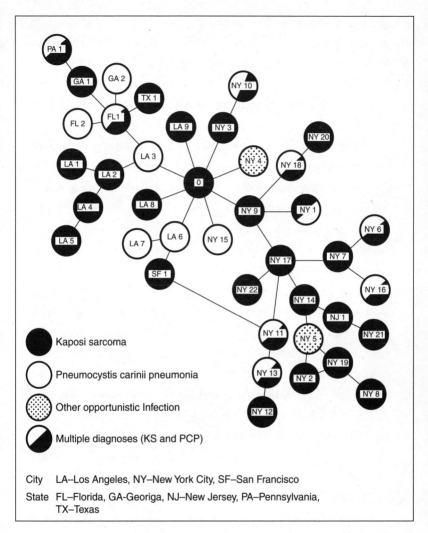

FIGURE 1 Diagram showing the sexual contacts of homosexual men with AIDs in cities in the US in the early 1980s. '0' represents patient zero.

Source: Figure 1 in Auerbach et al. American Journal of Medicine 76: 487–492. 1984.

the at-risk group and six months later haemophiliacs (who require regular infusions of blood plasma to control their bleeding tendency) were also on the list. When in July 1982 Haitians living in the US were suggested as the possible source of the disease, these supposed high-risk groups became known as the '4-H Club'—homosexuals, haemophiliacs, heroin addicts, and Haitians.

As long as the epidemic was confined to these specific groups the general public felt protected but all that changed between December 1982 and January 1983 when in rapid succession a child who had received multiple blood transfusions developed AIDS, cases of possible mother-to-child transmission were identified, and AIDS was reported in female sexual partners of bisexual men with AIDS. Now no one could deny that AIDS was spreading to the general population. This was confirmed in 1984 when two task forces sent to central Africa found AIDS cases of both sexes filling the hospitals. They described a massive, ongoing epidemic in central Africa spreading via heterosexual contact.

The media had a field day promoting scare stories until 'fear of AIDS' became a disease in its own right. Headlines like 'Exterminate gays' and 'Place AIDS victims in quarantine' fuelled stigmatization and victimization, and members of the high-risk groups, already subject to sexual, social, and racial prejudices, became scapegoats. All too commonly, children with AIDS were excluded from school, adults lost their jobs and homes, and families were subject to verbal and even physical abuse. Gay rights groups and AIDS charities worked hard to inform and educate, slowly redressing the balance. And the death of film star and heart-throb Rock Hudson from AIDS in 1985 did much to change public perception of the disease by 'giving AIDS a face.'[2]

Despite wild press speculation regarding the possible cause of AIDS, in May 1983 scientists at the Pasteur Institute in Paris led by Luc Montagnier and Françoise Barré-Sinoussi isolated a new virus from an AIDS sufferer. They called it LAV for lymphadenopathy-associated virus. Then in April 1984 workers at the National Cancer Institute in the US headed by Robert Gallo also announced that they had isolated 'the virus that causes AIDS', calling it HTLV III (for human T lymphotropic virus III). So began the 'great Franco-American virus war'[3]—the controversy over who had actually discovered the virus (soon called HIV for human immunodeficiency virus). Although this international dispute officially ended in March 1987 when Presidents Reagan and Chirac jointly announced a resolution by declaring co-discovery, in reality it rumbled on until 2008 when the Nobel Prize Committee decided to award the most prestigious prize in science to the French team—Montagnier and Barré-Sinoussi. Most scientists felt that right had finally prevailed.

This unfortunate saga should not overshadow the unprecedented speed of events: the causative virus was identified in less than three years of the first AIDS report, and shortly thereafter the genome was sequenced and clinical tests developed. Finally the disease could be diagnosed with confidence, virus carriers identified, and the spread via contaminated blood and blood products prevented.

* * *

At the time of the first AIDS report I was working in an immunology research unit at University College Hospital, London, where we, like others, were intrigued and horrified in equal measure by the rapidly unfolding series of events. We set up a collaborative research group that eventually identified the CD4 receptor molecule that HIV uses to infect its target cells—T lymphocytes. Naively, I assumed that the first descriptions of AIDS represented the beginning of the epidemic, but others were wiser. With the characterization of the virus in 1985, groups of evolutionary biologists around the world immediately started a search for its origin. They were asking: where had HIV come from? how had it first infected humans? and why had it spread so widely? In addressing these questions, scientists have scoured the world for specimens and utilized state-of-the-art techniques to unravel the strange and complex history of HIV in its most intricate details. Gratifyingly, these scientists have worked in a spirit of amicable scientific collaboration, and together they have found the answers.

This book traces their fascinating twenty-year quest—at once a tale of scientific endeavour and a detective story. It recounts the painstaking research that eventually unravelled how, when, and where HIV first infected humans, and how and why one particular type of HIV then spread globally. It seems appropriate to begin this book by outlining the convincing evidence that AIDS is indeed caused by HIV—the virus that has now invaded virtually every country in the world, infecting 60–80 million people and killing at least 25 million of them.

HIV/AIDS Timeline 1981–1987[4, 5]

1981—108 AIDS cases reported in US

June—Five gay men in Los Angeles reported with severe immunodeficiency.

July—Eight gay men in New York reported with Kaposi's sarcoma (KS).

December—Cases of AIDS reported in intravenous drug users in the US.

The first AIDS cases reported in UK.

1982—593 AIDS cases and 243 deaths in US

June—a cluster of AIDS cases in California suggests an infectious agent.

July—AIDS identified in haemophiliacs and among Haitians living in the US.

Acquired Immune Deficiency Syndrome (AIDS) officially adopted as the name of the new disease.

December—A 20-month-old multiply-transfused child dies of AIDS.

AIDS reported in infants suggesting mother-to-child transmission. AIDS reported in several European countries.

1983—1,972 AIDS cases and 759 deaths in US

January—AIDS reported in female sexual partners of men with AIDS.

March—Members of high-risk groups asked not to donate blood in US.

May—French scientists report isolation of a virus, LAV, from an AIDS lymph gland.

October—European and American AIDS task force sent to Africa to investigate.

September—People at risk of AIDS requested not to donate blood in UK.

November—WHO report AIDS cases in US, Canada, fifteen European countries, Haiti, Zaire, seven South American countries, and Australia.

1984—6,993 AIDS cases and 3,342 deaths in US

April—US scientists announce the isolation of AIDS-associated HTLV-III.

July—Ongoing AIDS epidemic reported in Rwanda and Zaire suggests heterosexual spread.

November—CD4 molecule on T cells identified as a receptor for HIV.

Publication of the genome sequence of LAV.

1985—10,000 AIDS cases and 4,942 deaths in US

January—Genome sequence of HTLV-III published.

March—The first AIDS test becomes available.

April—The first International AIDS Conference is held in Atlanta, US.

April—Report of mother-to-child transmission of HIV through breast feeding.

October—All UK blood transfusion centres begin routine testing for HIV.

Actor Rock Hudson dies of AIDS.

1986—28,098 AIDS cases and 15,757 deaths in US

May—Human Immunodeficiency Virus becomes the official name for the AIDS virus.

September—The first clinical trial of the drug zidovudine to treat HIV infection.

1987—40,051 AIDS cases and 23,165 deaths in US

March—Zidovudine approved for use in AIDS.

Presidents Reagan and Chirac sign an agreement over the discovery of HIV.

1

The Puzzle of HIV-1

In 2008 Luc Montagnier and Françoise Barré-Sinoussi from the Pasteur Institute in Paris were awarded the Nobel Prize in Medicine for their discovery of the AIDS virus now known as human immunodeficiency virus (HIV). Perhaps the Nobel Prize Committee was rather over-cautious in waiting over twenty years to honour the discoverers, but back in 1983 it was not immediately obvious that LAV, as the French team initially called the virus, was the cause of AIDS. They had undoubtedly isolated a new type of virus from a lymph gland of an AIDS victim, but it could have been the *consequence* rather than the *cause* of AIDS.

Everyone carries a number of viruses that persist in the body for life and are kept under control by a healthy immune system. With severe immunodeficiency these viruses often reactivate to cause opportunistic infections, and so they are much easier to isolate from tissues of those with AIDS. With the possibility that LAV could just be a passenger virus, many scientists initially reserved judgement over its causative link to AIDS. They were cautiously waiting for formal proof.

Right from the start the main opposition to the growing conviction that HIV causes AIDS was led by Peter Duesberg, a virologist from the University of California, Berkeley, US, and an expert in retroviruses, the virus family to which HIV belongs. He was vociferous in his opposition, speaking out at scientific meetings, writing extensively in scientific and lay press, and then setting out his 'AIDS denialist' arguments in detail in a book called *Inventing the AIDS Virus* published in 1996.[1] His arguments and the counter-arguments are worth summarizing here because his theories have not only misled individuals infected with HIV who were desperately looking for an alternative to the stark reality of their plight, but have also profoundly influenced public health policies. Most prominently, the South African government under Thabo Mbeki (president from 1999 to 2008), which had been advised by Duesberg, denied that AIDS caused by HIV was spreading in their country, and refused people the lifesaving treatment with anti-retroviral drugs they so desperately needed. This issue caused great concern in the early 2000s and resurfaced in late 2008 when scientists from Harvard University, US, published the results of a study on AIDS in South Africa. They estimated that between the years 2000 and 2005, 330,000 people in South Africa died unnecessarily from AIDS. Furthermore, during the same time period 35,000 babies were born with HIV infection that could have been prevented if their mothers had been provided with antiretroviral drugs. The scientists calculated that the total loss to South Africa was a massive 3.8 million person-years.[2] Duesberg's voice was immediately raised in protest. In a scientific paper published online in 2009 (but later retracted by the publisher because of its public health implications) he repeated his argument that HIV does not cause AIDS, concluding that Mbeki's decision to withhold antiretroviral drugs to those who were HIV positive had not caused the catastrophic death toll due to HIV.[3]

Initially Duesberg backed the theory that widespread use of recreational drugs known as poppers by gay men and the intravenous drugs taken by habitual users poisoned the immune system, leading to the profound immunodeficiency of AIDS. For haemophiliacs and blood transfusion-related AIDS he invoked immune overload, stressing that a unit of blood contains a large quantity of foreign protein that could equally well poison the immune system. He pointed out that half of all those given a blood transfusion for whatever reason die within a year of receiving the infusion, implying that consequently it was no surprise that so many haemophiliacs treated regularly with blood products were dying.

On the huge epidemic in Africa, Duesberg stated that 'African AIDS is not a specific disease, but a battery of previously known and thus totally unspecific diseases.'[4] According to his theory, Africans were dying of what they had always died of—malnutrition and common infections like gastroenteritis, pneumonia, and tuberculosis. In his opinion this was unrelated to HIV that was an ancient infection in Africa where it was harmlessly passed from mother to child.

Now that the case for HIV as the cause of AIDS has been proven to the satisfaction of the scientific community for over twenty years, Duesberg holds to his views and still has a following, albeit substantially diminished. Although he concedes that HIV and AIDS coexist in the West and target the same risk groups in the population, he insists that the former does not cause the latter. He believes that 'HIV is a harmless passenger virus'[5], and that scientists under pressure to come up with the answer to the spreading plague have convicted an innocent virus. Apparently at one point he even offered to inject himself with HIV to prove his point.[6]

A certain amount of scepticism in science is healthy, so when Duesberg first declared that HIV as the cause of AIDS did not fulfil the classic Koch's postulates, a set of criteria that should be met in order to prove that an organism causes a specific disease, most scientists agreed with him. HIV was recently discovered and it takes time to accumulate the evidence, but as study after study indicated a causal relationship between HIV and AIDS, Duesberg stuck to his guns.

Robert Koch, a German scientist who, along with Louis Pasteur, is often dubbed the Father of Bacteriology, set out his now famous postulates in the 1890s as follows:[7]

- The parasite [or microbe] occurs in every case of the disease in question and under circumstances that can account for the pathological changes and clinical course of the disease.
- It occurs in no other disease as a fortuitous and non-pathogenic parasite.
- After being fully isolated from the body and repeatedly grown in pure culture, it can induce the disease anew.

Koch, who isolated the first human pathogenic bacterium, *Bacillus anthracis*, in 1877, admitted that these postulates had limitations and would not all apply to every microbe. Bearing in mind that they were written before viruses were discovered, most scientists agree that if they are to be useful and relevant today they must move with the times. They should be revised as new knowledge and technologies dictate, as, indeed, they have been. Rather than going through the time-consuming and sometimes very difficult process of isolating a microbe from every case of a particular infectious disease, most scientists now accept indirect evidence of the infection such as finding antibodies against the microbe in the blood. These markers of infection can be very useful after the emergence of a new infectious disease such as, for instance, the epidemic of SARS (severe acute respiratory syndrome) that hit the world in 2003. Once a coronavirus was isolated from a case of SARS and an antibody test developed, screening of the relevant population showed that only those who had suffered from SARS had antibodies to this new coronavirus, thus incriminating it as the cause of the new disease.

The advent of molecular probes in the 1980s promised new, highly sensitive methods for detecting microbes in clinical samples without actually isolating them. In particular, a technique called the polymerase chain reaction (commonly known as PCR) invented by American chemist, Kary Mullis from Cetus Corporation, California, provided a highly sensitive way of amplifying specific DNA sequences. This has revolutionized the study of molecular biology, and in 1993 Mullis received the Nobel Prize in Chemistry for his invention. Since the PCR can detect tiny amounts of a specific genetic sequence and then amplify it up to workable levels, it was quickly utilized for identifying viruses, not least for detecting HIV in clinical samples.

* * *

Briefly considering each of Koch's postulates in turn for the case of HIV as the cause of AIDS as Duesberg has done, postulate one states that the microbe must be present in every case of the disease. Admittedly for HIV and AIDS at first this was a difficult call. The virus could not be isolated from all cases of AIDS as it was technically difficult to do so. However, once reliable tests for HIV antibodies became available these proved positive in the vast majority of suspected AIDS cases. But the presence of antibodies is indirect evidence of an infection, and Duesberg argued that it only denoted a past infection that had been eliminated rather than a persistent, ongoing infection. Everyone agreed that HIV, just like flu or measles viruses, caused an acute illness with flu-like symptoms called acute retroviral syndrome when it first infected a person, but in Duesberg's opinion the virus was then eliminated by the antibodies this generated, so preventing further disease.

When PCR testing for HIV in the blood was introduced, it gave positive results in virtually everyone with suspected AIDS. Duesberg then conceded that a low level of virus may persist in some cases, but pointed out that most people who were HIV positive by PCR did not have AIDS, and so concluded that HIV was a harmless passenger. Certainly far more people have positive HIV antibody and PCR tests than have AIDS. Early studies in the US followed two groups of gay men with the same risk factors for AIDS apart from HIV status. They soon showed that only those who were HIV positive went on to develop AIDS. When doctors calculated the lag period between HIV infection and the onset of AIDS to be between six and fifteen years, the reason for so many apparently healthy HIV positive people became clear.

Postulate one also states that the infection must account for the pathological changes seen in the disease. Proving this is complicated by the fact that HIV infection per se does not kill but causes a severe immunodeficiency that allows a whole gamut of other microbes to flourish and eventually kill in untreated cases. Virtually everyone now believes that HIV kills only indirectly but is nevertheless essential for the development of AIDS in a previously healthy person. However, the fact that AIDS victims suffer from a myriad of opportunistic infections means that the symptoms and the underlying pathological changes, are extremely variable. For this reason the first definition of AIDS published in 1982 by the Centers for Disease Control in Atlanta, US, was inevitably imprecise, consisting of a long list of clinical conditions, such as *pneumocystis* pneumonia (caused by *P carinii*, now called *Pneumocystis jirovecii*), thrush, and shingles, occurring in a person with no known cause for diminished resistance to disease.[8] However, early immunological studies on gay men soon identified the key pathological event that occurs during the asymptomatic phase of HIV infection. This is declining numbers of CD4 T cells in the blood and their depletion in lymph glands and other organs. CD4 T cells are pivotal to generating effective immunity against invading pathogens, and HIV specifically targets this population of T cells, infecting and destroying an estimated 1–2 billion of them daily, and in doing so producing up to 100 billion new viruses. In untreated HIV infections the destruction of CD4 T cells eventually outstrips the body's ability to regenerate them, and when the numbers decline to below the critical level of 200 per microlitre of blood, opportunistic microbes invade and AIDS develops. In the light of this, the case definition of AIDS was revised in 1993 to include a blood CD4 T cell count of less than 200 per microlitre in an HIV positive person.[9] Today this HIV-mediated destruction of CD4 T cells can be halted, and the onset of AIDS prevented, with drugs that specifically target HIV. When these are administered, the virus load in the body goes down and will only rise again and cause AIDS if a mutation renders the virus resistant to the drugs or the patient stops taking them—a clear indicator that HIV causes AIDS. Perversely though, Duesberg has added this lifesaving treatment to his list of toxic drugs that actually induce AIDS because, he says, it is toxic to cells of the immune system.[10]

In the pre-AIDS era clinical immunologists were well acquainted with severe immunodeficiency and its associated opportunistic infections occurring in children born with congenital immune disorders. They also saw it in adults with an underlying illness that suppresses immunity like leukaemia or lymphoma, in those undergoing treatment for cancer, and in people taking drugs specifically to suppress their immunity to prevent rejection of a transplanted organ. Very occasionally immunologists recognized an AIDS-like illness in a person without any recognizable underlying cause, and this they attributed to the late (adult) onset of a congenital immune disorder. These cases continued to crop up after AIDS was recognized and for a time they caused confusion by being labelled 'HIV negative AIDS'—a boost for Duesberg's campaign. However, once it was clear that sufferers were not in any of the risk groups for HIV/AIDS, and that the number of these cases was not rising, most were happy with the label immunologists had given them.

Postulate two, that the microbe cannot be found in any other disease, is again tricky to interpret for viruses like HIV that persist in the body for life. These viruses are readily detected with sensitive techniques like PCR, and obviously during a lifetime of infection with persistent viruses, a person will suffer from many other unrelated infections. For instance, after a childhood infection, lifelong carriage of several herpes viruses, including the cold sore and chickenpox viruses, is the norm, so the fact that they may be isolated from people suffering from flu or the common cold does not mean that they are the cause of these ailments. The same logic applies to HIV.

Obtaining direct proof to satisfy postulate three by inoculating the pure culture-grown microbe in question into an uninfected host to reproduce the same disease has always been problematic with human diseases/microbes. Notwithstanding famous (and infamous) experimenters of yester-year such as John Hunter, who injected himself with the microbes that cause syphilis and gonor-rhoea, and Edward Jenner, who inoculated a child with cowpox followed by live smallpox virus, clearly these days this direct approach is not ethical. It is sometimes possible to reproduce the disease in an animal model infected with the microbe under test, like, for example, flu virus that will infect mice and ferrets, but this is by no means always the case. Indeed some microbes, such as those that cause leprosy, typhoid fever, and diphtheria, cannot even be propagated in the laboratory, while others like hepatitis A and B viruses, and HIV, do not reliably cause disease in any experi-mental animal species. However, for HIV, a number of tragic 'nat-ural experiments' has provided the answer to postulate three.

First, mother-to-child transmission of the virus first recognized in the early 1980s, occurs in around a quarter of pregnancies where the HIV infected mother does not take prophylactic anti-retroviral drugs. Molecular analysis of HIV isolates from mothers and their HIV positive babies shows around 97 per cent identity in genome sequences. This is around the same level of identity found between two viruses taken from the same person, thus indicating that both viruses came from the same source. Furthermore, only babies of HIV positive mothers who are HIV positive themselves go on to develop AIDS; those that do not acquire the virus from their mothers remain healthy.

Second, early in the AIDS pandemic many haemophiliacs were infected with the virus by infusions of blood-clotting factor VIII that had been concentrated from the blood of several thousand blood donors, some of whom were HIV positive. UK records show quite clearly that the outbreak of HIV in haemophiliacs began in 1979, and came from contaminated factor VIII imported from the US. The outbreak ended after the problem came to light in 1986 when the imports were stopped. During these eight years, 1,227 of the 6,278 haemophiliacs living in the UK acquired HIV, and between 1984 and 1991 the death rate for this HIV positive group was ten times higher than in a comparable HIV negative group; 85 per cent of these deaths were due to AIDS.[11]

Third, a small cluster of related cases was uncovered in 1990 when, to the horror of the American public, Kimberly Bergalis from Florida, US, a young woman with no apparent risk behaviours for acquiring HIV, who was nevertheless dying of AIDS at the time, publically declared that she had been infected with HIV by her dentist.[12] The dentist in question, Dr David Acer, tested HIV positive in 1986 and developed AIDS in 1987. He continued to practise dentistry until 1989. After this revelation, all Acer's patients were offered an HIV test and over 1,100 accepted. Ten tested positive and of these, five, including Bergalis, reported no high-risk behaviour for HIV acquisition other than invasive dental work performed by the dentist. Molecular analysis of their virus isolates showed that all five patients (and one other with 'indeterminate risk behaviour'), had HIV isolates that were so closely related to the dentist's and each other's viruses that they must have derived from a single source—most likely the dentist.

If these three incidents are not enough to convince that HIV causes AIDS (and apparently for Duesberg they are not), then the fourth, the accidental infection of three laboratory workers reported in 1994, is clear proof.[13] One research technician tested HIV positive on routine screening for people working with the virus. A second reported puncturing their skin while using a centrifuge previously used for concentrating HIV samples, and a third person was accidentally sprayed on the face with concentrated HIV. One of the three developed an AIDS-defining illness, *pneumocystis* pneumonia, sixty-eight months after the accident, and all three had markedly low CD4 T cell counts at the time the cases were reported in the medical press. None had risk behaviours for acquiring HIV infection, and only one of the three was given antiretroviral drugs prior to symptoms developing. All three cases were infected with a pure laboratory clone of HIV, and the same clone was later recovered from their blood, so indicating that the laboratory strain was the cause of their symptoms.

Thus by the early 1990s all but a few were content to accept this as proof that HIV causes AIDS and move on. We are left with the AIDS denialists who, by definition, 'reject the objective reality [in order] to sustain a flawed, hurtful, and ultimately dangerous belief system.'[14]

* * *

HIV is a virus unlike any other. It works by stealth, silently entering the body and wiping out the very immune defences that have specifically evolved to fight such invaders. Without modern drug treatments it eventually kills virtually everyone it infects, but only after a period of ten years or so. At first it shows no outward signs of its presence and this is the key to its success. Those living with HIV, unaware of the virus within, get on with their daily lives and in so doing unwittingly spread the virus to others. The end game only begins when the immune system is so weakened that all manner of microbes can invade and flourish, thus causing the terrible symptoms of AIDS. So what is this virus and how does it work?

HIV belongs to the retrovirus family, a large and ancient group of viruses that infect many vertebrate species. These viruses are generally harmless in their natural hosts but if transferred to another species they may cause a variety of diseases ranging from cancer to anaemia and immune deficiency. When HIV was first identified in 1983 only two other human retroviruses had already been discovered. Both of these were identified by Robert Gallo and co-workers at the National Institute of Cancer, Bethesda, US, while hunting for viruses that cause human cancers. He concentrated on leukaemia, developing methods for propagating the malignant blood cells in culture with the help of growth factors and for detecting reverse transcriptase, an enzyme uniquely produced by growing retroviruses. In 1981 all his hard work paid off when he detected reverse transcriptase in a single culture of cells from a leukaemic patient. Gallo isolated human T lymphotropic virus (HTLV) I from the patient's malignant cells and showed that this retrovirus causes the rare blood disorder, adult T cell leukaemia. This discovery was followed by the isolation of a second human retrovirus, HTLV II, but so far this has no disease associations. Gallo's discoveries, and the technical advances that made them possible, set the scene for the isolation of HIV by Barré-Sinoussi and Montagnier shortly afterwards and for the identification of several related viruses that followed.

The history of retroviruses began over 100 years ago. In 1908 two Danish scientists, Wilhelm Ellermann and Oluf Bang, transmitted leukaemia from one chicken to another with a tumour cell extract that had been filtered to exclude whole cells and bacteria. This experiment did not cause much interest until 1911 when Peyton Rous, working in the US, reported similar tumour transfer using a cell-free extract of a solid tumour from a chicken. The reports predated the characterization of viruses and so, although work continued on these 'filterable agents', other scientists were sceptical of their very existence. Rous was only awarded the Nobel Prize for his seminal discovery in 1966, some fifty years after the event. In the meantime a 'milk agent' (now known to be mouse mammary tumour virus) that increased the incidence of cancer in pups from mothers with breast cancer was discovered by fellow American, John Bittner. Then in 1936 and in 1951 Ludwig Gross from New York published evidence of a mouse leukaemia virus. All these animal tumour viruses, at the time called oncoviruses, later turned out to belong to the retrovirus family, but this only became apparent after their remarkable method of replication was elucidated in the 1970s.

* * *

Retroviruses, in common with several other virus families, including those to which flu and measles viruses belong, carry their genetic material as RNA rather than DNA. But the retrovirus life cycle has a unique step that allows these viruses to colonize their respective hosts for life. Each virus particle contains two copies of the RNA genome along with the reverse transcriptase enzyme, which enables retroviruses to convert their RNA genome into DNA. During the unravelling of this replication cycle reverse transcriptase was discovered independently by American scientists Howard Temin and David Baltimore. The implications of this discovery appeared to belie the central dogma of molecular biology in which genetic information flowed exclusively from DNA to RNA to protein, and so it was initially met with disbelief. However, the evidence was overwhelming, and in recognition of this scientific breakthrough, Temin and Baltimore shared the Nobel Prize for Medicine in 1975.

When a retrovirus infects a cell, its reverse transcriptase converts the viral RNA genome into double-stranded DNA, and another enzyme carried in the virus particle called integrase then catalyses the joining, or integration, of the viral DNA copy into that host cell's DNA chain. Now part of the cellular genome, the virus is protected from immune attack and remains there for the life of the cell, being replicated along with cellular DNA and passed on to daughter cells.

The integration process effectively archives retroviral genomes for the life of the infected cell, and if the virus gains access to germ cells then it will pass from one generation to the next ad infinitum. This latter scenario may seem rather far-fetched but when the human genome was sequenced it revealed a remarkable 96,000 retrovirus-like elements occupying around 8 per cent of the entire genome. Nobody really knows what they are doing there but scientists speculate that they are fossils—the remains of ancient virus infections. Maybe some of them caused plagues like HIV/AIDS, and if so then perhaps in several thousand years' time a fossilized HIV will be found fixed in the human genome.

* * *

With the exception of RNA viruses, all other living organisms carry their genetic material as DNA. The two molecules are structurally similar, each built from four nucleotides, or bases, that make up the letters of the genetic alphabet. In DNA these are adenine (A), cytosine (C), thymine (T), and guanine (G), with A binding to T and G to C in the double helix. RNA structure differs from DNA in that the thymine is replaced with uracil (U), giving the base pairs AU and GC. Genes consist of unique sequences of As, Cs, Gs, and Ts (or Us in RNA), with each group of three adjacent letters coding for one of the twenty essential amino acids, the building blocks from which proteins are made.

Every time a cell divides, the entire length of its DNA, consisting of 3×10^9 base pairs in humans, is copied, with one copy destined for each daughter cell. The fidelity of the copying process is vital for the survival of the species since a change of just one letter in the genetic code may alter a protein in a detrimental or even lethal way. For this reason, DNA replication is tightly controlled to ensure that new strands have an identical nucleotide sequence to the old. Before a cell actually divides, new DNA strands are proof-read and any mistakes corrected; thus the number of errors, or mutations, passed on to daughter cells is extremely small, at around one in two hundred million nucleotides per year.

Compared to humans, viruses have a high mutation rate, and for RNA viruses this is particularly high at around one in every thousand nucleotides per year. This is because there is no proof-reading step during replication of the RNA genome. Also, the generation time of viruses is very short, sometimes just a matter of a few hours, with thousands of new viruses produced at each cycle. Many viral offspring will carry mutations, some of which will be deleterious, and some have no effect at all. Just a few will be beneficial to the virus, maybe because they increase its replication rate, enhance its ability to evade the immune response, or allow it to spread more effectively between hosts. Any of these benefits increase the 'fitness' of a virus, such that its offspring would soon come to dominate the viral population. As we will see in future chapters, rapid mutation has been one of the keys to HIV's success.

* * *

Traditionally, uncovering the evolutionary history of a species has involved studying fossilized remains, radiocarbon dating samples from them, and using this information to construct an evolutionary, or phylogenetic, tree—a branching diagram showing the relationships between different species. In a tree, such as the primate tree depicted in Figure 2, each junction, or node, indicates the most recent common ancestor, and the length of the branches emerging from a junction give an estimate of the time that has passed since the species diverged. In the case of humans, prior to the 1960s scientists were able to piece together an evolutionary tree of sorts from the few ancient hominid fossils discovered over the previous few decades. However, large gaps made it difficult to calculate exactly when we diverged from our nearest living relative, the chimpanzee, the best estimate being around 15 million years ago. Since the 1960s these fossil-based calculations have been augmented by molecular methods for estimating evolutionary time. Called the molecular clock, the technique is based on the premise that any gene mutations occur at a roughly constant rate. So, just like the rate of radioactive decay that is used to radiocarbon-date fossils, although mutations occur randomly, over long periods of time the ticking of the molecular clock is reasonably regular. From this it follows that the more similar the DNA sequences of a given gene from two different species are, the more closely the species are related to each other. Additionally, quantifying the difference between the two gene sequences provides an estimate of the time to their most recent common ancestor. For example, to calculate the date of divergence of humans and chimpanzees the molecular clock was first calibrated using DNA sequences from primate species whose divergence date was already known fairly accurately from fossil records. Then, comparing a large number of human and chimpanzee gene sequences, scientists came up with a new estimate of between just six and seven million years ago. This figure, being so at odds with the previous estimate, came as a shock at the time but it actually now agrees with the fossil record that has increased significantly since the 1960s. Thus, the recently calculated one per cent difference between the entire human and chimpanzee genomes is in line with our very slow mutation rate over six to seven million years of divergence.

Since viruses do not generally leave fossil records, the molecular clock is the only way to uncover their history. Although in most organisms the mutation rate is so low that this technique is only useful for investigating their ancient history, viruses are different. With a mutation rate around a million times higher than that of humans we can more easily delve into a virus's recent past and even study its evolution over short periods of time. Indeed, as we will see in later chapters, for viruses like HIV the molecular clock is more

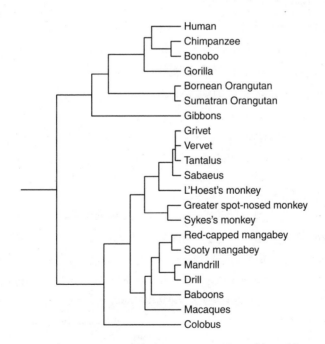

FIGURE 2 Evolutionary tree including representative old world apes and monkey species.

Source: Perelman et al. Plos genetics 7(3): e1001342. 2011.

accurate for the recent rather than the ancient past. This is partly because their habit of mixing and matching parts of their genomes with other viruses eventually tends to obscure the picture.

Flu virus is a good example of a rapidly changing virus. Its RNA genome is constantly mutating in its natural host, that is wild birds, particularly water fowl. Scientists regularly monitor this to detect any new strains with the potential to jump to humans and cause a pandemic. Below is a small part of a sequence from a flu virus gene showing how it mutated between 1933 and 1985:[15]

1933—CTCTGTACCTGCATCGCGC
1934—CTCTGTACCTGC**G**TCGCG**T**
1942—CTCTG**C**ACCTGC**T**TCGCG**C**
1947—CTCTG**C**ACCTGC**T**TCGCG**C**
1950—CTC**CG C**ACCTGC**T**TC**T**CG**A**
1977—CTC**CG C**ACCTGC**T**TC**G**CG**A**
1980—CTC**CG C**AA**C**TGC**T**TC**G**CG**A**
1984—CTC**CG C**AA**C**TGC**T**TC**A**CG**A**
1985—CTC**CG C**AA**C**TGC**T**TC**A**CG**A**

* * *

Prior to the 1980s, viruses were classified into families and subfamilies according to their shape, size, and genome type (RNA or DNA), but with the advent of genome sequencing everything changed. The first complete human virus genome sequence was published in 1985 revealing vital clues about the virus's evolutionary history. As more sequences followed, the relationships between different viruses became clearer and this information has been used to revise and refine their classification. On this basis, retroviruses were divided into genera (alpha-epsilon), all with the same overall structure. They have just three major genes called *gag*, *pol*, and *env*, that code for virus coat proteins, the viral enzymes and the virus envelope proteins respectively. We will meet these genes again in later chapters.

The HIVs are all grouped together in the lentivirus subfamily. The name means 'slow virus' because if the members cause disease at all it is generally only after a long lag period. When HIV was first isolated, only a few lentiviruses were known, and its nearest relative was the visna virus of sheep (Figure 3). This led to speculation, outlined in chapter 2, about how visna virus might have jumped to humans to become HIV. But when the first simian immunodeficiency virus was identified as the cause of simian AIDS in 1985 and added to the lentivirus subfamily, things became a little clearer. Now around forty simian immunodeficiency viruses have been isolated, all of which are more closely related to the HIVs than is visna virus. By convention these viruses are referred to as SIV followed by the abbreviated name of the monkey from which they were isolated—for example, the natural host of SIV_{agm} is the African green monkey and SIV_{cpz} is from chimpanzees. Uncovering the mysterious origin of the first SIVs shows just how useful the molecular clock and the construction of evolutionary trees can be.

* * *

Soon after the first description of AIDS in 1981, American scientists at the New England Regional Primate Research Center, Boston, noticed a similar disease affecting their captive macaques, a primate species that originates from Asia. Just like AIDS sufferers, these animals developed enlarged lymph glands, diarrhoea, weight loss, and muscle wasting, and suffered from lymphomas as well as severe opportunistic infections including *pneumocystis*

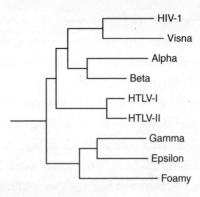

FIGURE 3 Evolutionary tree showing the lentiviruses HIV-1 and visna in relation to the other retrovirus genera.

Source: Figure 1 in Bailes et al in The molecular epidemiology of human viruses. Ed Thomas Leitner. Kluwer Academic Press. 2002.

pneumonia, tuberculosis, thrush, cytomegalovirus, and other herpesvirus infections. The disease invariably proved fatal. Also mirroring AIDS in humans, the animals' lymphocyte function was poor and many had low lymphocyte counts.[16, 17] The newly recognized syndrome became known as simian AIDS.

At the New England Center an increase in death rate in macaques was first noted in 1980, with one third of their colony of Taiwanese rock macaques (*Macaca cyclopsis*) dying in that year alone. Interestingly, tests on samples stored from post-mortem examinations revealed that some macaques had died of simian AIDS as early as 1970. Since these early cases occurred in animals that had been obtained from the California Primate Center, Davis, the suspicion was that one or more of them had been infected prior to transport to Boston, and that the root of the problem lay in California.[18] Indeed, when the scientists in California looked back at their records, they found that immunodeficiency–related illnesses in their macaques actually predated the first description of AIDS in humans, with four separate outbreaks occurring between 1969 and 1981.

Naturally, the description of simian AIDS precipitated a hunt for the culprit virus, and in 1985, scientists at the New England Primate Center isolated a simian immunodeficiency virus (specifically SIV$_{mac}$), from four rhesus macaques (*Macaca mulatta*) with simian AIDS.[19] This virus induced simian AIDS within weeks when inoculated into healthy macaques. So here was a direct cause and effect relationship between virus and disease that immediately fulfilled Koch's postulates. But that was not the end of the story. Several animals which later developed simian AIDS or their ancestors had been unwittingly shipped around the US from one primate centre to another and were sometimes housed along with other primate species in large outdoor 'corrals' containing fifty or more animals. Here the virus could have jumped to them from any co-housed species, perhaps via transfer of blood or saliva during fights that regularly break out between monkeys kept in such large groups. So it was feasible that macaques were not the natural host for SIV$_{mac}$.

Until the late 1980s simian AIDS mainly affected rhesus macaques but then outbreaks of the disease occurred in a related species, the stump-tailed macaque (*Macaca arctoides*) at primate centres in California and also at the Yerkes National Primate Research Center in Atlanta, where they had received the animals from the California Center. Subsequently another virus, SIV$_{stm}$, was isolated from these sick animals,[20] but the identity of the natural host(s) of these SIVs still remained a mystery.

In the last twenty years an intensive hunt for retroviruses carried by Old World primates has turned up around forty different SIVs. However, these viruses were all isolated from wild African primates, with none identified in wild Asian primates. It seems that Asian primates, including macaques, do not carry SIVs in the wild, thus strengthening the theory that captive macaques had picked up SIV from African primates within the primate centres.

An important clue to the true identity of SIV_{mac} came in 1986 when scientists noted that SIV_{mac} was very similar to a retrovirus found in healthy, captive sooty mangabey monkeys (*Cercocebus atys*), a species native to West Africa. However, they were cautious until 1989 when a new retrovirus was isolated from both captive and wild sooty mangabeys. This provided sure evidence that this mangabey species was the natural host of the virus.[21] The genome sequence of this virus, called SIV_{smm}, turned out to be very closely related to SIV_{mac}. and SIV_{stm}. Indeed the 12 per cent difference between the sequences of one particular gene from the two viruses is no greater than that found between isolates of SIV_{smm} from two naturally infected wild sooty mangabeys. This level of similarity showed that the two viruses had diverged from each other recently, probably in the late 1960s or early 1970s.

It turns out that wild-caught West African mangabeys were imported to the US on many occasions over a fifty-year period ending in 1968. This timing fits with SIV_{smm} jumping species from its natural host to macaques in the primate centres to produce SIV_{mac} and SIV_{stm}. Just four primate centres in the US imported and housed colonies of sooty mangabeys: The California National Primate Research Center; New Iberia Research Center, Louisiana; Yerkes National Primate Research Center; and Tulane National Primate Research Center, Louisiana. In order to get to the bottom of the mystery surrounding the origin of SIV_{mac}, scientists carried out an extensive molecular study on SIV_{smm} isolates from sooty mangabeys housed at these centres over the previous thirty years. Genome sequences from 84 SIV_{smm} isolates were used to construct an evolutionary tree to identify their relationship to each other and uncover the origins of the macaque viruses SIV_{stm} and SIV_{mac}.[22] This revealed that at least nine of the sooty mangabeys from West Africa were naturally infected with SIV_{smm} at the time of importation to the US. Over the thirty-year period, these nine viruses had spread naturally in the sooty mangabey colonies at the four centres. Scientists pinpointed two of these viruses that had jumped from sooty mangabeys to macaques, both at the California National Primate Research Center, where they became the ancestors of SIV_{mac} and SIV_{stm}. Once in the macaques, SIV_{smm} spread easily within the colony by various means: sexual contact, mother-to-child transfer, and possibly through blood contamination during fights. The viruses must have then replicated virtually unchecked in their new host so that by the 1980s when simian AIDS first came to light several different subtypes of the virus had already evolved and were co-circulating in the primate centres.

Given that there must have been many opportunities for this type of cross-species transmission between sooty mangabays and macaques housed together over a fifty-year period, the fact that only two such incidents occurred suggests that natural interactions between caged animals do not generally lead to interspecies transfer of the virus. In fact scientists traced the origins of SIV_{mac} and SIV_{stm} back to the 1960s when some rather more invasive work was going on—Carleton Gajdusek was experimenting with kuru at the primate centre in California.[23]

Kuru is a human, neurodegenerative disease, very like the new variant Creutzfelt-Jacob disease (CJD) that recently spread from cows to humans in the UK via infectious proteins called prions. However, kuru only affected the remote Fore-speaking tribe in Papua New Guinea,[24] and the infectious agent, now also known to be a prion, was spread among members of the tribe through the custom of eating their dead. Fortunately, now that the practice of cannibalism has died out, the disease has finally become extinct. At the time of its discovery in 1957 kuru was thought to result from a slow virus infection, and Gajdusek and his team were trying to reproduce it experimentally by inoculating a variety of primates including mangabeys and macaques with blood and tissues from cases of kuru. The material was injected both into the bloodstream and the brain of the animals, and 'infected' material from these injected animals, presumably sometimes containing SIV_{smm}, was then used to try to infect further healthy recipients. So although this procedure only aided SIV_{smm} to jump once from a sooty mangabey to a macaque, with more than 1,500 animals used in the experiments overall it is not surprising that SIV_{smm} was soon rife among macaques at the centre. When the kuru experiments ended with apparently healthy animals, SIV_{smm} infected macaques were sold on to the New England Center, thereby unwittingly spreading the virus to this primate colony.

The only other incident of SIV_{smm} jumping to macaques occurred in the 1980s during similarly invasive studies, this time on leprosy at the primate centre in Tulane.[25] Sooty mangabeys are among the few animals known to be naturally infected with the leprosy bacterium, *Mycobacterium leprae*, and in these experiments scientists were attempting to transmit the bacterium to other primates including macaques. Blood and lepromatous material from naturally infected sooty mangabeys were injected into the skin and/or the bloodstream of rhesus macaques, on one occasion transferring SIV_{smm} at the same time. This seeded the virus that later caused an outbreak of simian AIDS at the Tulane Center. Interestingly, virus-contaminated lepromatous material was also passed between sooty mangabeys and, although most of these animals were already naturally infected with SIV_{smm}, on one occasion this produced a double, or super-, infection with an additional virus strain. Within a month this animal harboured a recombinant virus made up of a mixture of genes from its own and the new strain's genomes, an indication of just how labile these viruses can be.

Although retroviruses commonly cause disease in non-natural hosts, the emergence of such a highly pathogenic strain of SIV_{mac} that caused simian AIDS in just a few weeks is unusual for a so-called slow virus. Indeed, SIV_{mac} is the only SIV that causes disease in macaques. When SIV_{smm} is transferred directly from sooty mangabeys to macaques, not all infected animals develop simian AIDS and some even clear the virus completely. This suggests that SIV_{smm} had changed during its residence in macaques, and scientists suspected that evolution of this highly pathogenic virus was the result of the unnatural routes of spread used in the kuru experiments. They suggest that inoculation of virus directly into the brain and bloodstream followed by serial passage from one susceptible animal to another may have selected for, and propagated, a particularly virulent strain.

The investigation into this man-made outbreak of simian AIDS concluded that some highly invasive experimental practices unwittingly transmitted an unknown infectious agent from one primate species to another. The transport and reuse of experimental animals complicated the issue and probably prevented identification of the ongoing problem of simian AIDS until the description of AIDS in humans around ten years later. Happily, with present-day legislation regarding animal experimentation in place in most countries, this unfortunate episode is unlikely to be repeated. However, the incident does have a positive side. SIV_{mac}

infection in macaques provides the best model system for investigating the pathogenesis of HIV infection and AIDS and for testing out potential antiretroviral agents and HIV vaccine candidates. Furthermore, the molecular detective work that unravelled the origin of SIV$_{mac}$ revealed viral diversity of the same magnitude as that seen in pandemic HIV-1 in humans, although, as we will see in the next chapter, this proved to be a much more complex puzzle.

2

Tracing HIV to its Roots

Peter Piot, a Belgian clinical microbiologist, was working at the Institute of Tropical Medicine in Antwerp when, in 1979, people first turned up at his clinic with unusual, what he terms 'weird', infections. He remembers that to begin with these were exclusively men and women with links to Africa—either Africans or Europeans who lived, or had lived, in Africa. Because of previous colonial links with Belgium most of these patients came from Zaire (previously the Belgian Congo and now the Democratic Republic of Congo (DRC)). One of these early cases that particularly sticks in Piot's mind was a Greek fisherman who lived and worked on the shores of Lake Tanganyika in east Zaire. He suffered from severe, life-threatening infections that eventually proved fatal. The autopsy findings really shocked Piot. The patient's internal organs were virtually destroyed by an atypical mycobacterial infection. These microbes are related to *Mycobacterium tuberculosis* but are common in the environment and generally harmless. To find them causing such widespread and devastating disease in a previously healthy person was perplexing to say the least. But, unknown to Piot, the fisherman had a severe immunodeficiency and, when HIV tests became available five years later, analysis of stored blood samples showed that he had HIV infection. However, back then Piot did not immediately make the connection between cases like this one and the first description of AIDS published in June 1981. The American reports referred exclusively to gay men with an immunodeficiency causing *Pneumocystis* pneumonia and/or Kaposi's sarcoma, while Piot and his colleagues were seeing unusual infections, but not *Pneumocystis* pneumonia or Kaposi's sarcoma, in heterosexuals, equally affecting men and women.

As part of his job at the Institute of Tropical Medicine, Piot ran a clinic for sexually transmitted diseases. Many gay men attended this clinic and in late 1981 he began to see men with the typical symptoms of AIDS, and most of these cases had visited the US recently. Only then did Piot make the connection between these two apparently unrelated epidemics, one in Africans and the other in gay men, and realized that they could have a single cause.

Around the same time Piot discovered that colleagues in Brussels were also seeing Africans with bizarre infections, and by 1982 he reckoned that around 100 such cases had been treated in Belgium. Since only a small minority of Africans could afford to get their medical care in Belgium, Piot realized that this was just the tip of the iceberg—there must be many more AIDS cases in Africa. He set about organizing a fact-finding mission to Zaire, but getting funding proved difficult, and it was 1983 before a team of European and American infectious disease specialists headed for Kinshasa, the capital of Zaire.

Piot had previously worked in the country. In 1976 as a young microbiologist he had been part of the team that investigated one of the first recorded Ebola virus outbreaks. This was in the remote village of Yambuku in the north-west of Zaire. Even so he was completely unprepared for what they saw there. In Mama Yemo Hospital, with 2,000 beds the largest and one of the best-equipped general hospitals in Sub-Saharan Africa, they found wards full of terminally ill young men and women. The commonest symptoms were weight loss and severe, persistent diarrhoea along with TB, Kaposi's sarcoma, and many other infections. Dr Kapita, the head of internal medicine, although not a specialist in infectious diseases, was alone among the medical staff in realizing that something unusual was afoot. He met the visiting team with a pile of patient files from affected cases, most of whom were already dead.

Back in 1983 there was no specific test for HIV. Even so Piot's team set up a laboratory in the University Hospital of Kinshasa where they performed simple blood-screening tests. Crucially, these revealed that the African patients had the same lack of CD4 T cells that had been reported in the first AIDS victims in the US, suggesting that they were all suffering from the same disease. At this point Piot had what he describes as an 'aha moment', suddenly realizing the likely extent of the pandemic and the human cost of it, and perhaps also anticipating his own personal role in combating it. In 1984 Piot teamed up with Jonathan Mann from the US Centers for Disease Control to set up Project SIDA (Syndrome d'Immuno-Déficience Aquise) in DRC, the first and largest AIDS research project in Africa. Then in 1995 Piot became head of the newly founded organization UNAIDS, remaining there until 2008.

Piot's report of the team's visit to Zaire was published in *The Lancet* in 1984 alongside a similar report from Kigali, capital of

Rwanda.[1,2] Together these clearly demonstrated that HIV was well established in central Africa where it affected both men and women and was spread by heterosexual contact. They also showed an annual incidence of AIDS in Kinshasa and Kigali that was much higher than in San Francisco or New York, thus dispelling any lingering notion that AIDS was a disease restricted to ethnic or sexual minority groups. By 1985 further studies in Kinshasa and Kigali demonstrated very high levels of HIV infection in female commercial sex workers and pinpointed this group as an important source for dissemination of the virus to a wider population.

*　*　*

The intense and sometimes unguarded publicity surrounding the reports on AIDS in Zaire and Rwanda ensured that the issue immediately became highly sensitive and politically charged. The reaction from African countries varied: some chose to ignore the threat while, as is common at the start of an epidemic, most found others to blame for its origin. Several regarded the whole thing as an attempt on the part of the West to blame Africa for the developing crisis on its own doorstep. However, for some countries the reports served as a wake-up call and their governments were ready to rise to the challenge. Foremost among these was Uganda where the term 'slim disease' was first coined for African AIDS. This differed clinically from AIDS in the West because the patients suffered from different opportunistic infections. The term 'slim disease' evocatively portrays the severe, chronic wasting disease that characterizes AIDS in Africa. First seen in the rural district of Rakai on the shores of Lake Victoria near the Ugandan-Tanzanian border in 1982, the disease was widespread by the time its description was published in 1985. To quote a typical patient history from the report:

In the first six months the patient experiences general malaise and intermittent fevers for which he may treat himself or receive asprin, chloroquine or chloramphenicol. In due course he develops loss of appetite.

In the next six months intermittent diarrhoea starts. There is gradual weight loss and the patient is pale. Most patients at this point in time rely on traditional healers, as to many the disease is attributed to witchcraft.

After one year the patient typically develops a maculopapular rash, which is very itchy, all over the body. The skin becomes ugly with hyperpigmented scars. There may be a cough, usually dry but sometimes productive. By this stage, sometimes earlier, the patient is so weak that, if taken to hospital, not much can be done to help him and death follows.[3]

Doctors investigating slim disease found that risk factors included having multiple sexual partners and previous sexually transmitted diseases. It affected both sexes equally leaving doctors in no doubt that it was sexually transmitted, and was caused by HIV. They suggested that the virus had been brought to Rakai by Tanzanian traders or soldiers and was thereafter spread by female commercial sex workers in a pattern that was to become familiar across Africa and beyond.

When all consenting patients admitted to fifteen hospitals throughout Uganda during one week in 1987 were tested for HIV, 42 per cent turned up positive.[4] Although these early HIV tests later proved to give erroneously high figures in blood samples from Africans, at the time that this figure was reported it did much to shock the world out of any complacency over the spreading HIV pandemic. In fact over 18 per cent of people in the Ugandan capital, Kampala, were HIV positive. Those infected were typically young, sexually active businessmen or male clerks who travelled frequently, had multiple sexual partners, and had previously suffered from sexually transmitted diseases. Homosexuality and intravenous drug use were not evident in this population. The report left no doubt that slim disease, and thus HIV, was flourishing in Uganda.

Similar reports soon followed from other African countries and, as the dust settled, it became clear that by 1987 HIV had invaded thirty-seven of the forty-seven African countries surveyed, of which Zaire, Rwanda, Burundi, Uganda, Zambia, and Tanzania were the worst affected. Spread to surrounding countries mainly followed major highways and trading routes. It was rapid and proved impossible to stop. Figures from the Kenyan capital, Nairobi, illustrate the explosive nature of an HIV epidemic and its introduction to the general population through commercial sex workers. In 1981 4 per cent of female commercial sex workers were HIV positive; this figure had risen to 61 per cent by 1985. In parallel, none of over 100 men with genital ulcers (suspected clients of sex workers) were HIV positive in 1981; by 1985 15 per cent were positive, by which time 2 per cent of pregnant women, representing the general population, were infected.[5, 6]

* * *

Remarkably, despite their proximity to high incidence areas and the rapid spread of HIV elsewhere, by the mid 1980s very few AIDS cases were reported from the West African countries of Senegal, Nigeria, Ghana, Mali, Sierra Leone, The Gambia, Guinea-Bissau, and Ivory Coast. Because it was clear that female sex workers acted as a source for HIV dissemination in Rwanda and Zaire, in 1985 doctors tested blood samples from a similar group of women in Senegal. Initially 7 per cent of Senegalese sex workers were found to be HIV positive although all were apparently healthy at the time. However, scientists found that the antibodies in their blood showed unusual reaction patterns, binding more strongly to the proteins of SIV_{mac} (the virus isolated from captive macaques in 1985) than those of HIV. This raised suspicions that a different type of virus might be circulating in West Africa,[7] and the race was on to identify it.

In 1986 Montagnier and co-workers in Paris isolated a new retrovirus from the blood from two West African AIDS sufferers. The investigation had begun a year earlier when a Portuguese scientist visited the Pasteur Institute in Paris to learn virus isolation techniques. She brought with her a blood sample from a 29-year-old man from Guinea-Bissau who had been unwell for two years and was currently being treated in the Egas Moniz Hospital in Lisbon. He had all the symptoms of AIDS but had repeatedly tested HIV antibody negative. Later in 1986, a similar HIV-negative patient was discovered at the Claude Bernard Hospital in Paris. This was a 32 year old man from the Cape Verde Islands, off the coast of Senegal, who had been treated for recurrent infections at the hospital since 1983.[8] Investigations showed that both patients had the same retrovirus in their blood. This turned out to be a new lentivirus which had a similar overall genome structure to the AIDS virus already identified and spreading in the US, Europe, and Central Africa, but paradoxically it was quite a different virus.

This new virus was subsequently isolated from many other AIDS sufferers and healthy people in West Africa. So it seemed that, like HIV, it could cause AIDS but could also remain as a silent infection for many years. The virus mirrored HIV in infecting CD4 T cells and primarily spreading by sexual intercourse or blood contact. However, it differed from HIV in some important features. First, analysis of its genome sequence showed that the virus was only distantly related to HIV, but was more closely related to SIV$_{mac}$. Second, the virus was less virulent than HIV in that it maintained a lower viral load in healthy carriers, had a lower rate of transmission to contacts, and sustained a longer lag period before the onset of AIDS. Indeed some of those infected never developed the symptoms of AIDS and went on to die from unrelated causes. These differences seem to account for the virus remaining local to West Africa. The new virus, initially called LAV-2, is now officially called HIV-2 to distinguish it from the original, more widespread virus, now designated HIV-1.

With the knowledge that HIV-2 was closely related to SIV$_{mac}$, the search for its origin concentrated on isolating novel SIVs from African primates. The hunt took place concurrently with the hunt for the ancestor of SIV$_{mac}$ in captive macaques (described in chapter 1). Rather surprisingly, the two stories rapidly converged. After SIV$_{smm}$ was isolated from captive and wild sooty mangabeys, it soon transpired that this virus was not only the ancestor of SIV$_{mac}$ but also of

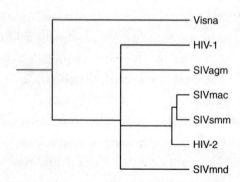

FIGURE 4 Evolutionary tree showing the relationship between Visna, HIV-1 and HIV-2 and the simian immunodeficiency viruses that had been isolated by 1989.

Source: figure 1 in Jin et al EMBO J 13: 2935–2947. 1994.

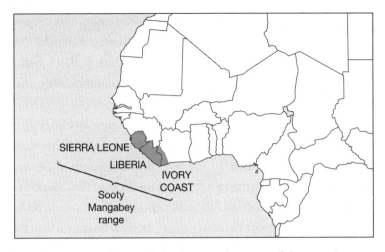

FIGURE 5 Map of West Africa showing the range of the sooty manga-bey monkey.

HIV-2. In fact, at the genetic level HIV-2 and SIV_{mac} are more closely related to each other than either is to HIV-1 (Figure 4). Comparing the sequences of viral proteins, SIV_{smm} and HIV-2 are between 62 and 87 per cent identical, a level of identity that indi-cates that the two viruses shared a common ancestor in the fairly recent past—perhaps as recently as 50–60 years ago.[9] This infor-mation implies that HIV-2 must have jumped from one species to the other, and since sooty mangabeys coexist with humans in West Africa, this theory is entirely plausible. The animal's range used to extend all along the west coast of Africa from the Casamance River in Senegal in the north to the Nzo/Sassandra River basin in the Ivory Coast in the south, the very region where HIV-2 is endemic. But with loss of forest habitat and bush-meat hunting taking their toll, wild sooty mangabeys are now restricted to Liberia, Sierra Leone and the western part of the Ivory Coast (Figure 5).

The jumping virus scenario provides two logical alternatives: either SIV_{smm} represents the ancestral virus that jumped from sooty mangabeys to humans or HIV-2 is the parent that jumped from humans to sooty mangabeys. To begin with, genome analysis of the existing virus isolates showed more genetic variability between individual HIV-2 genomes than among those of SIV_{smm}. This suggested that the virus had evolved for longer in humans, so favouring the human to monkey transfer theory. However, when more human and sooty mangabey viruses were added to the evolutionary tree both viruses were seen to be equally diverse. It is now accepted that the sooty mangabey is the natural host for the virus since infection is more common in this species. SIV_{smm} is carried by around 50 per cent of these animals in the wild whereas the highest level of HIV-2 infection recorded in humans in any country is in the region of 8–10 per cent. Furthermore, SIV_{smm} infection appears to be non-pathogenic in sooty mangabeys, suggesting a long association with its host, whereas, as we have seen, HIV-2 can cause AIDS in humans.

The most probable route for virus transfer from sooty mangabey to human is through contact with blood from an infected animal. As sooty mangabeys are commonly hunted for bush-meat in West Africa this certainly provides the opportunity for blood contact via a bite or a cut during the process of killing and butchering the animals. Also, orphaned animals are often kept as household pets in the area, and in this situation again a bite could transmit the virus. Support for this comes from an interesting study on pet animals in Liberia and Sierra Leone in which SIV_{smm} isolates were generally found to be quite genetically divergent from each other. Surprisingly though, they appear to be more closely related to HIV-2 isolates from the same geographical location. Equally surprising, SIV_{smm} isolates from sooty mangabeys kept as pets in Liberia and Sierra Leone were most closely related to HIV-2 virus isolates from people living in the same area.[10]

As soon as HIV-2 was discovered, researchers began to track back to find out when and where it first infected the inhabitants of West Africa. Stored blood samples from healthy people in the area revealed the first evidence of HIV-2 infection in the 1960s. The very low level of infection at that time suggested that its introduction to the population was recent, perhaps just prior to 1960. Later studies identified Guinea-Bissau as the country with the highest level of infection, and within this country the highest prevalence was in the north-east in the rural area around Canchungo. A survey carried out here in 1992 showed a rate of HIV-2 infection around 8 per cent, with only one in a thousand (0.1 per cent) being HIV-1 positive.[11] This area of the country was therefore seen as the epicentre of the epidemic.

These surveys also uncovered some intriguing epidemiological differences between HIV-1 and HIV-2 in Africa. Whereas HIV-1 mainly infected young, sexually active adults, in Bissau, the capital of Guinea-Bissau, the highest levels of HIV-2 infection were seen in people aged between 50 and 69 in whom it reached around 15 per cent. The prevalence of HIV-1 in the same group was just 0.5 per cent.[12] Of course, this peak of HIV-2 infection in older people could have been an artefact caused by a high death rate among young infected people. However, the particular risk factors for HIV-2 infection found in this older age group suggest a different explanation. Guinea-Bissau, formerly Portuguese Guinea, was a Portuguese colony until 1974 when the country gained self-rule after a war of independence lasting eleven years. Because the risk factors for HIV-2 infection mostly related to sexual transfer, with the additional risk for men of being in the army, scientists pointed the finger at the war of independence as the likely event that kick-started the epidemic. They speculated that the influx of Portuguese soldiers and the chaos of war with its inevitable increase in migrant workers and commercial sex would allow a sexually transmitted virus that had hitherto remained at a very low level in the community to reach epidemic proportions. The cohort of 50–69 year olds studied in 2000 would have been in their 20s and 30s during the war years and therefore at their most sexually active and consequently most likely to acquire and spread the virus.

A change in medical practices during the war years may also have played a part in spreading the virus via infected blood. First, large vaccination and treatment programmes for diseases like TB and sleeping sickness were organized by army doctors. Second, blood transfusion became more widely available to treat war victims and the general public. While vaccination may have spread the virus via the reuse of non-sterilized needles, which was common practice at the time, this was compounded by the increased use of blood transfusion that unwittingly provided another mode of virus transmission. A case in point is that of a 57–year-old Portuguese woman whose husband served in the Portuguese army and whose family lived in Guinea-Bissau from 1960 to 1974. They then returned to Portugal where in 1991 she was found by chance to be HIV-2 positive. She had received a blood transfusion in 1967 after suffering a spontaneous abortion, and in the absence of any other risk behaviours, this seemed to be the most likely source of the infection. Her husband and children, one of whom was born after the transfusion, had not picked up the virus and she was still symptom free when the case was reported in 1995.[13] Thus clearly the virus had entered the blood supply line in Guinea-Bissau by 1967.

Not surprisingly Portugal was the first country outside West Africa to report cases of HIV-2-related AIDS, and even now around 12 per cent of AIDS in Portugal is caused by this virus. Most sufferers are either from Guinea-Bissau or are Europeans who visited or worked in the country. Members of the Portuguese armed forces were particularly at risk, so lending support to the theory that the circumstances of war aided virus spread.

* * *

Eight different groups of HIV-2 (named A-H) have now been isolated. When placed in the evolutionary tree with related retroviruses these strains are interspersed among SIV_{smm} isolates (Figure 6). This shows that they are each more closely related to a certain strain of SIV_{smm} than to other HIV-2 groups. This being the case the eight HIV-2 groups could not have evolved from a single source, or even one from another, after jumping from sooty mangabeys to humans. Therefore, surprising as it may seem, they must each represent a separate transmission event.

To date only two HIV-2 groups, A and B, have succeeded in spreading; the others have each been isolated from just one individual. To unravel the evolutionary history of these two groups scientists compared the genome sequences of thirty-three viruses with known dates of isolation to estimate the date of their most recent common ancestors. For all group A viruses this turned out to be sometime around 1940 and for all group B viruses around 1945. Thus, since these virus ancestors must have evolved in the sooty mangabey, these dates represent the last possible time at which they could have jumped from monkeys to humans. The same scientists then calculated the approximate date of the most recent common ancestor of A and B strains in the sooty mangabey

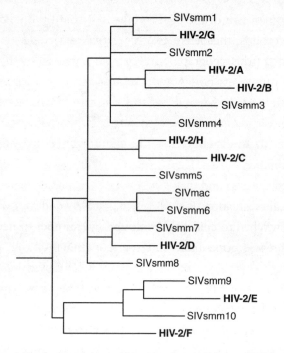

FIGURE 6 Evolutionary tree showing the position of HIV-2 groups A-H interspersed by SIV$_{smm}$ isolates.

Source: Figure 5 in Sharp and Hahn in Cold Spring Harb. Perspect. Med. Cold Spring Harbor Laboratory Press. 2011.

Note: The order of clustering of viruses differs among trees derived from different viral genes, reflecting recombination between viruses circulating in sooty mangabeys (this tree was obtained using part of the gag gene). When all trees are considered, it becomes apparent that each group of HIV-2 must have originated from a separate introduction to humans.

at some time near the end of the 19th century, thus providing us with the earliest possible date for their individual transfer to humans.[14]

Exactly where within the sooty managabey's range the eight strains of HIV-2 jumped to humans is not known, although a large study on free-ranging sooty mangabeys in the Taï Forest, Ivory Coast, identified viruses in these animals that cluster so closely with five of the eight groups, including the epidemic A and B groups, that it is possible that these viruses jumped to humans in this geographical area.[15] However, if this is correct then it is not clear how A and B group viruses spread to Guinea-Bissau from their origin in the forests of Ivory Coast.

Genetic analysis of virus isolates from the epidemic area in Guinea-Bissau shows a very slow rate of virus growth during the 1940s and early 1950s. This suggests that perhaps just a few viruses reached the area and that at first they only spread slowly among the local population. But all this changed around 1955 when the virus switched to epidemic mode and the number of new infections grew exponentially.[16] Indeed, between 1955 and 1970 the estimated growth rate of HIV-2 in Guinea-Bissau was greater than that of HIV-1 in west central Africa. The timing of this dramatic expansion of HIV-2 coincided with the war of independence in Guinea-Bissau, so corroborating the suggestion that this was the critical event to kick-start its rapid local spread.

As it turned out, tracing HIV-2 back to its origin proved relatively easy, and importantly, this work was key to eventually identifying the origin of HIV-1. The revelation that HIV-2's direct ancestor was SIV from the sooty mangabey stimulated scientists to isolate SIVs from many more African primate species, and this work led eventually to the identification of the ancestors of HIV-1.

*   *   *

By the 1980s many felt that HIV-1 had its origin in west central Africa and had been imported to the US in the 1970s, but there was no real evidence for this and no consensus. Several crazy theories hit the headlines, including totally unscientific ideas suggesting that HIV, in true biblical fashion, was dispensed by an angry god or that it had arrived from outer space. Others suggested that the virus was developed for germ warfare either in the US or by the Nazis during World War II.[17] However, a few scientists put forward the serious proposal that the virus originated in the US or Europe where it had been endemic for a long time. They suggested that the infectious nature of AIDS had escaped notice until the 1980s because the virus had struggled to survive in a generally non-promiscuous society where intravenous drug use was virtually unknown. One suggestion that put the origin of HIV firmly in Europe was that HIV-1 arose from visna virus. This virus, HIV's closest known relative before the discovery of the SIVs in the mid 1980s (see Figure 3), was first isolated from sheep in 1949, but had been causing outbreaks of encephalitis and pneumonia in sheep in Iceland since the 1930s.[18]

Assuming that HIV-1 really did arise in the US or Europe then the trigger for its epidemic spread was presumed to be the socio-cultural changes consequent on the sexual revolution of the 1960s and the gay liberation movement in the 1970s. Certainly as gay bars, discos, bathhouses, and sex tourism proliferated so the incidence of STDs rose with both syphilis and hepatitis B virus infections tripling in gay men during the 1970s.

Doctors and researchers looking for clues relating to the place of origin of HIV-1 pursued three lines of enquiry: they scoured the medical literature prior to the first description of AIDS for cases of fatal immunodeficiency and/or Kaposi's sarcoma that satisfied the early AIDS definition; they searched out old collections of blood samples and tested them for HIV; and they collected and analysed HIV-1 genomes from around the world. Each approach proved interesting and informative but it was the combination of all three that finally provided the answer.

Many medical case reports were found that *could* have represented early HIV infections that had gone unrecognized before the landmark AIDS report in 1981.[19] One of the earliest American examples was a previously healthy 28-year-old man from Memphis, Tennessee, who was diagnosed with viral pneumonia in February 1952. From then on he suffered recurrent infections until his death in December of the same year. Autopsy provided a diagnosis of concurrent cytomegalovirus and *Pneumocystis* infections—typical of AIDS cases in the US. In Europe possible AIDS cases from the 1970s were mostly in young, sexually active gay men who had visited the US or Haiti, suggesting that the virus had arrived in Europe from the West via international gay sexual networks. Interestingly, the investigation also uncovered several possible cases in Europeans who had lived in Central Africa in the 1970s. One such was a 47-year-old Danish woman doctor who worked as a surgeon in Northern Zaire from 1972 to 1975 and then in Kinshasa until 1977 when she returned to Denmark. From 1976 onwards she suffered from persistent diarrhoea and later developed enlarged lymph glands. She died of *Pneumocystis* pneumonia in December 1977.[20]

In France and Belgium, as we have already seen, many Africans with AIDS were treated in the early 1980s and retrospective analysis pushed this influx back to 1977. In August of that year a 34-year-old African woman from Kinshasa brought her 3-month-old daughter to hospital in Louvain, Belgium. Two of the woman's children had died at the age of 6 months from severe infections and the third had suffered from persistent thrush since birth. While this child was receiving treatment the mother became unwell and was admitted to the hospital. She suffered from weight loss, generalized enlarged lymph glands and a respiratory infection, and her blood lymphocyte function was found to be low. Between September 1977 and January 1978 she contracted a series of severe infections and when her condition deteriorated she decided to return to

Kinshasa where she died in February 1978.[21] All these cases are tantalizing but, unfortunately, with no stored samples suitable for HIV testing, the diagnosis of AIDS remains speculative.

The earliest AIDS case in the US shown to be HIV-1 antibody positive was that of a 15-year-old American from St Louis, Missouri, who was heterosexual, had never travelled beyond the immediate area of St Louis, and had never had a blood transfusion. He had been sexually active for several years prior to 1968 when he first consulted doctors about persistent swelling of his lower body. His condition deteriorated progressively until he died in 1969. Disseminated Kaposi's sarcoma was diagnosed at autopsy. Blood and tissue samples that had been frozen in 1969 were tested in 1988 and proved positive for HIV antibodies. This result apparently established that HIV-1 had been in the US since at least 1968.[22] Disappointingly though, these results were later questioned and without reliable genome sequences from the infecting virus for evolutionary studies, this case could provide no further information on the past history of HIV-1.

Turning to Africa, it was no surprise that very few cases of unusual infections were reported in the medical literature before the first description of AIDS, since fatal infectious diseases in young people were all too commonplace. Thus it is likely that the earliest AIDS patients with opportunistic infections would have gone unnoticed. When I met with Dr Kapita some sixteen years after Piot headed the fact-finding taskforce to the Mama Yemo Hospital in 1983, he still clearly recalled the first case of AIDS he had seen at the hospital in 1978. This was a nurse from Haiti, and since her Congolese husband was healthy, Kapita surmised that she and other professionally trained Haitians who came to the country in the 1960s and 1970s may have brought the virus with them.

In contrast to the paucity of information on unusual infections, changes in the incidence or nature of Kaposi's sarcoma were likely to be recognized in Central Africa where it was, and still is, a common and distinctive tumour. Prior to the AIDS pandemic, Kaposi's sarcoma was most prevalent in Zaire, Rwanda, Burundi, Cameroon, Tanzania, and Uganda where it generally affected adult men. The tumour was described as indolent, or slow-growing. Many sufferers survived for ten years or more after diagnosis, although a more aggressive type of Kaposi's sarcoma was occasionally seen in African children. Indolent Kaposi's sarcoma was also seen in the US and Europe but it was extremely rare, mainly confined to elderly men of Mediterranean or Jewish descent. In the US the incidence of Kaposi's sarcoma began to rise in the late 1970s co-incident with a change from the classic indolent disease to the more aggressive tumour now seen in association with HIV-1 infection in gay men. Reports from Africa noted a rising incidence of Kaposi's sarcoma beginning around 1980, and in 1983 Anne Bailey, a surgeon from Lusaka, Zambia, identified a clinically atypical, more aggressive type of Kaposi's sarcoma among her patients.[23] In an extensive series of patients from Zambia and Uganda, where a recent rise had also been seen, she found 96 per cent of the atypical, aggressive Kaposi's sarcoma cases were HIV-1 antibody positive compared to 17 per cent of the classic, indolent cases. This study was reported in 1985 when 20 per cent of healthy Ugandans used as controls were HIV-1 positive compared to just 2 per cent of the Zambian controls, a result that reflected the recent arrival of HIV-1 in Zambia, but its widespread invasion of Uganda.[24]

* * *

Eventually this thorough trawl of the medical literature with subsequent review of dozens of possible AIDS cases turned up just two that tested HIV-1 positive. Both were from Europe and both had served in their country's navy; they are now known as the Manchester sailor and the Norwegian sailor. The case of the Manchester sailor was first reported in the medical literature in 1960.[25] Previously healthy, he was 25 years old when he first became ill in December 1958. As far as is known he was heterosexual, and did not use intravenous drugs. He spent his national service in the UK Royal Navy from 1955 to 1957 and was said to have travelled abroad. However, on thorough investigation it transpired that apart from a brief trip to Gibraltar, with a possible day trip to Tangiers, he was stationed in England for the duration. At first his symptoms were suggestive of generalized TB but, as treatment for this was ineffective and no *Mycobacterium tuberculosis* could be detected in his sputum, the drugs were discontinued. His condition continued to worsen and he became severely wasted with large, painful herpesvirus ulcers on his face and genital area. Finally he developed pneumonia that did not respond to antibiotics and he died in September 1959. Autopsy revealed *Pneumocystis* pneumonia and cytomegalovirus infections in his lungs. Samples of the man's organs were preserved in formalin and stored.

In the late 1980s PCR amplification of virus sequences from formalin fixed material became technically possible and the virologists at the University of Manchester set up the procedure in order to test the Manchester sailor's stored samples. They used similar tissue samples from a man of the same age who had died in a road-traffic accident in 1959 as a negative control, an HIV-1 infected cell line as a positive control, and coded the samples so that the investigator was blind to their identity. They must have been delighted when they decoded the results and found that only the positive control and four other samples were positive—those from the sailor's kidney, bone marrow, spleen, and pharynx. They reported these positive results in 1990, thus laying claim to the first recognized case of AIDS in the world.[26]

The Norwegian sailor was married with three children and was therefore assumed to be heterosexual. He served in the Royal Norwegian Navy from 1961 to 1965, during which time he travelled widely. Between 1961 and 1962 he sailed along the West African coast stopping off at several ports in Nigeria and later visiting Asia, Europe, Canada, the Caribbean, and East Africa. While in the navy he twice contracted sexually transmitted diseases. He became unwell in 1966, aged 20, with joint and muscle pains, enlarged lymph glands, a skin rash and recurrent respiratory infections. An autoimmune disease was diagnosed for which he received treatment and his condition remained stable until 1975. He then developed lung disease and progressive neurological problems with dementia. He died in April 1976. The sailor's wife first became ill in 1967 at the age of 24 with recurrent infections including persistent oral thrush. From 1973 onwards she lost weight and suffered from encephalitis. In 1976 acute leukaemia was diagnosed and she died in December 1976. Of the couple's three daughters, the two eldest remained healthy while the youngest, born in 1967, suffered from recurrent severe infections from the age of 2 until her death from chickenpox in 1976. Blood and tissue samples from all three cases were stored, and tests carried out in 1971 showed that they all had low lymphocyte function. Initial HIV tests in 1986 proved negative but retesting using more sensitive methods in 1988 found all three family members to be positive.[27] Since no other cases of HIV infection or AIDS have been uncovered in Norway from the 1960s the most likely scenario for this tragic family drama is that the sailor acquired HIV-1 during one of his visits to Africa. He then passed the virus to his wife through sexual intercourse and it later infected the youngest daughter either while *in utero* or shortly after birth, perhaps via breast milk.

* * *

In parallel with the literature trawl, the search for stored collections of blood samples that might have proved valuable for detecting early HIV infections was equally thorough but no HIV antibody positive samples were found in the US, Haiti, or Europe prior to the 1970s. Furthermore, disappointingly few archived sample collections had survived in west central Africa. This was particularly true of the DRC where all frozen samples were lost during times of unrest and civil war when electrical failures were frequent and unavoidable. Fortunately however, a few collections of African blood samples from past studies that were stored abroad have survived and have proved invaluable. These show that the prevalence of HIV-1 infection in Kinshasa had risen to 5 per cent by 1985 and it has remained around this level ever since, showing that the virus has reached equilibrium in the population and its level has stabilized.

In contrast to this urban situation, when, in 1988, 659 stored samples from the village of Yambuku in north-east Zaire taken at the time of the Ebola virus outbreak in 1976 were HIV-1 tested, just five (0.8 per cent) were positive. By 1985–6 three of these HIV-1 positive villagers had died of illnesses suggestive of AIDS. However, HIV testing in the same region at that time gave exactly the same result as ten years earlier, telling us that while the HIV epidemic was spreading in the urban population of Kinshasa it had not yet taken off in this rural community.[28]

The largest collection of samples from a variety of African countries, taken between 1959 and 1982 for population genetic studies and containing over 1,000 frozen blood samples, was found safely stored in a freezer in the US. Of these samples, 818 dated from 1959. When these were tested for HIV-1, 92 per cent initially gave positive results, but, mindful of the high rate of false positive results found in African samples using early HIV anti-body tests, particularly those stored for long periods, scientists re-tested samples with the highest level of antibody by two other tests. Ultimately, only one sample was unequivocally HIV-1 positive in all the tests. All that is known about the donor of the positive sample, designated L70, is that he was an adult Bantu male who was living in Leopoldville (now Kinshasa) in 1959. There was no evidence of HIV-1 in samples in the collection from rural areas of the Belgian Congo, again stressing the urban focus of the early epidemic.[29] Thus it seems that HIV-1 has been present in Central Africa since 1959, around twenty-five years before it was first isolated.

*   *   *

With two apparently authenticated cases of HIV-1 infection dating from 1959, (one from the UK and one from Central Africa), and another in Norway from the early 1960s, it was imperative to find out how closely they were related to each other. This required recovering genome sequences from the infecting viruses and placing them in the retrovirus evolutionary tree. This was expected to help to solve the puzzle of the time and place of origin of HIV-1.

*   *   *

From the mid 1980s onwards scientists had been collecting and analysing HIV isolates from across the globe, and sending the sequences to the HIV database at Los Alamos National Laboratory, US, where they are collated. It soon became apparent that HIV-1 shows a remarkably high degree of genetic diversity. In fact, individual isolates form part of a spectrum of viruses in which no two are identical but all are sufficiently closely related to each other to be obviously derived from a common ancestor. However, in 1990 a new type of HIV-1 was isolated in Piot's laboratory from an AIDS patient from the Cameroon.[30] This new virus is geographically restricted to the Cameroon and neighbouring countries where it is responsible for between 1 and 5 per cent of all HIV-1 infections. Comparison of the amino acid sequence of its proteins with pandemic HIV-1 showed only 50 per cent identity, indicating that this was a new, rare type of HIV-1. This virus is now called HIV-1 group O, with the pandemic strain being HIV group M. In 1998 a third type of HIV-1 was found, also in a Cameroonian AIDS sufferer. Named HIV-1 group N, this virus is extremely rare and also restricted to West Africa.[31] Retrospectively, rational meanings have been given to these group names: M for major, O for outlier and N for non-M, non-O. Because of their level of diversity and their positions in the evolutionary tree interspersed between SIVs, scientists are convinced that the three groups of HIV-1 (M, O and N) were introduced separately into humans.

*   *   *

In 1997 partial HIV-1 genome sequences were obtained from stored lymph gland material from the Norwegian sailor and his daughter, although no viral sequences could be amplified from his wife's tissues. Rather surprisingly, father and daughter turned out to be infected with an HIV-1 group O virus, presumably acquired while the sailor was visiting West African ports in 1961–2.[32] Given the degree of diversity between HIV-1 group O and M protein sequences, this finding could explain the initial failure to detect HIV-1 antibodies in blood samples from the family.

The massive global diaspora of HIV-1 group M, combined with its high mutation rate, has led over a relatively short time span to the evolution of nine subtypes or clades (A–D, F–H, J, K) that differ from each other by 25–35 per cent in the amino acid sequences of their envelope proteins. The progenitors of all these subtypes apparently diverged nearly simultaneously in what has been delightfully termed 'a starburst' (Figure 7a). To add to this complexity there are also a variety of sub-subtypes and recombinant viruses in circulation. The latter have arisen by recombination of two or more HIV-1 genomes inside an individual with multiple infections. Such an event turns out to be quite common; indeed, the reason that there are no subtypes called E and I is because the original viruses with these designations were found to be recombinants themselves. E was composed of parts of subtypes A and E and I predominantly of subtypes A, G, H, and K. Recombinant viruses now account for around 18 per cent of all HIV-1 group M infections, and with virus evolution continuing apace their number will inevitably increase. As we will see in future chapters, their discovery was very important in unravelling the history of the HIVs. Fortunately though, understanding the ins and outs of the complexity of the virus subtypes is not our goal here: we are only concerned with how molecular and evolutionary analyses of viruses finally pinned down the place of origin of the pandemic.

In general HIV-1 group M subtypes are distributed geographically (Figure 7b), so allowing the progress of the pandemic to be traced. On a worldwide scale HIV-1 group M subtypes A, B, and C are the commonest, with subtype C accounting for almost half of all infections. Subgroup A predominates in Central and Eastern Africa and Eastern Europe; B is the main subtype in the US, Western and Central Europe, and Australia, while C is responsible for most

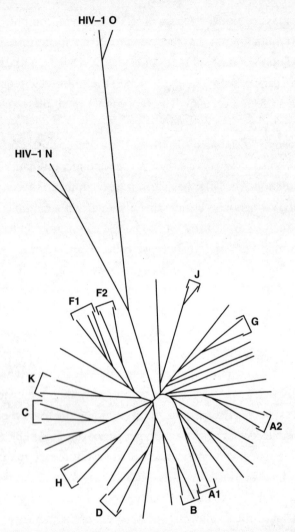

FIGURE 7a Diagram of the HIV-1 group M 'starburst' showing the evolutionary relationships between the HIV-1 groups and subtypes. The unlabelled lines represent recombinant forms.

Source: Figure 1 in Buonaguro et al J Virol. 81: 10209–10219. 2007.

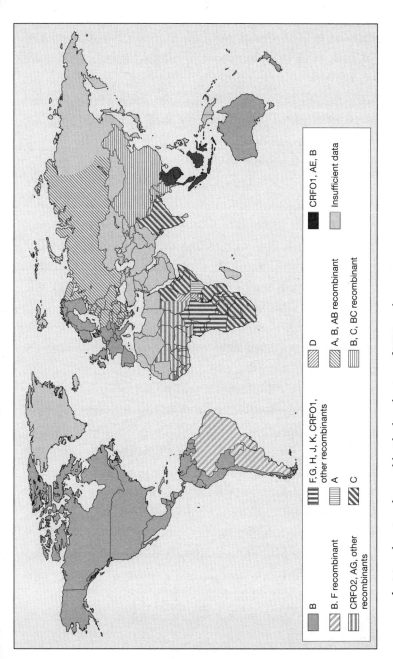

FIGURE 7b Map showing the worldwide distribution of HIV-1 subtypes.

Legend:

- B
- B. F recombinant
- CRFO2, AG, other recombinants
- F,G, H, J, K, CRFO1, other recombinants
- A
- C
- D
- A, B, AB recombinant
- B, C, BC recombinant
- CRFO1, AE, B
- Insufficient data

infections in South Africa and India. However, it is most striking that virtually all HIV-1 subtypes and many recombinant forms are circulating in west central Africa,[33] suggesting that the virus has been resident and evolving there for quite some time, but no one can say exactly how long unless some 'fossil' viruses can be found.

Because of its importance in tracking the evolutionary history of HIV-1, the Manchester sailor's tissue samples were sent to the Aaron Diamond AIDS Research Center, New York University, US, where scientists succeeded in amplifying viral sequences. They then sent these to the HIV database at Los Alamos National Laboratory where they were slotted into a comprehensive HIV-1 evolutionary tree. Unfortunately, from then on the case that had the potential to uncover HIV-1's mysterious past began to unravel.

The sailor's virus belonged to HIV-1 M subtype B, the most common subtype in the US and Europe. Worryingly though, the genome sequence fitted into the evolutionary tree among the most recent HIV-1's of this subtype, meaning that it was indistinguishable from the B subtypes currently circulating in the US and Europe. Given the long time span since the infection occurred, and the rapid rate of virus evolution, this seemed highly unlikely. Further, when they checked the tissue type of the samples they found that the tissues were derived from two separate individuals. Reporting this information in the journal Nature in 1995, David Ho and colleague Tuofu Zhu said that this finding raised 'the spectre of specimen contamination'.[34]

With confirmation of the modernity of the genome sequence from other experts, it is now accepted that contamination with a laboratory strain of HIV-1 must have occurred within the Manchester laboratory—a cautionary tale for any would-be PCR technologists.

With the Norwegian sailor and his family infected with the non-pandemic HIV-1 group O virus and the exclusion of the Manchester sailor from the field by 1995, the HIV-1 positive blood sample, L70 from Kinshasa, was left standing alone as the only hope for pinpointing the epicentre of the pandemic. Miraculously, in 1998, after nearly forty years of storage and with only a minute quantity of material to work with, Zhu and Ho managed to amplify short sequences of the HIV-1 genome from this sample. They identified it as an HIV-1 group M virus which to this day remains the oldest such genome in existence.[35] Fortunately the virus, now called ZR59, is not a complex recombinant, which might have caused problems in placing it in an evolutionary tree. In fact it displays features of both subtype B and D viruses. As it turns out these two subtypes are more closely related to each other than to the other subtypes and ZR59 represents an ancestral sequence for these subtypes fitting into the HIV-1 group M evolutionary tree close to the B/D common ancestor. With a single stroke this position in the evolutionary tree rules out the possibility that HIV-1 subtype B was present in Europe in the 1930s, let alone Europe being the place of origin of the AIDS pandemic.

The position of ZR59 in the evolutionary tree suggests that west central Africa, and particularly Kinshasa, was the epicentre of the HIV-1 M pandemic. This suggestion is strongly supported by studies on more recent virus isolates from this area as well as other geographic areas. Several studies have now documented an unprecedented level of genetic diversity in HIV-1 group M viruses from Kinshasa. All known subtypes are co-circulating there with subtype A predominating. Not only is there such a high degree of diversity in Kinshasa but there are also many complex recombinant forms. This all indicates that HIV-1 has probably been circulating in the city for longer than anywhere else in the world. Therefore, considering all the evidence, west central Africa, and particularly Kinshasa, had finally been identified as the most likely epicentre of the pandemic. Consequently this is where scientists concentrated their search for the origin of HIV-1 group M. We follow this search in the next chapter.

3

The Primate Connection

By the mid 1990s it was clear that the epicentre of the HIV-1 pandemic was in west central Africa, in the region encompassing the DRC and Cameroon. But even when it became apparent that the virus had jumped to humans in this area on at least three separate occasions, the identity of its animal reservoir remained a mystery. Obviously it was important to find this missing link, not least in the hope of preventing this lethal virus from jumping again. But although the hunt for HIV-2's direct ancestor, SIV_{smm}, recounted in chapter 2 was fairly rapidly rewarding, it took over twenty years to come up with the definitive answer for HIV-1.

Many different primate species live in the vast tropical forests of DRC , Gabon, the Republic of Congo, and the Cameroon, and several pieces of evidence pointed to an SIV carried by one of these species as the direct ancestor of HIV-1. First, although SIVs from only two species had been identified by 1985, as more and more primate viruses were isolated (the figure reached 20 by the late 1990s) it transpired that they were all lentiviruses with a genome structure similar to HIV-1. Also, they were all related to HIV-1 genetically, indicating that they had derived from a common ancestor at some time in the past. Second, just like the sooty mangabey that carries the direct ancestor to HIV-2, chimpanzees, bonobos, mountain and lowland gorillas, baboons, drills, and mandrills, and many smaller monkey species, are all commonly hunted for food, with their young often being kept as pets. This provides a possible transmission route for SIVs from primates to humans via blood contact, and once it was generally accepted that HIV-2 had jumped from sooty mangabeys to humans on several occasions, either via a bite from a pet animal or during the hunting and preparation of bush-meat, most believed that HIV-1 groups M, O, and P had done the same, but from an as yet unknown primate carrier.

Determined to uncover the origin of HIV-1, scientists intensified their search for viruses infecting African primates in the hope of finding an SIV that was so closely related to HIV-1 that it must be its direct ancestor. The work involved testing primates' blood for antibodies that reacted with HIV or SIV proteins as a marker of infection with a related virus. But, practically speaking, capturing and bleeding these animals on a large scale in the wild is just not possible, so scientists initially opted for testing captive animals from zoos and primate centres around the world. This turned up disappointingly few new SIVs, adding just two more to the evolutionary tree of primate lentiviruses by 1989. These viruses, SIV_{agm} from African green monkeys (*Ceropithecus aethiops*) and SIV_{mnd} from the mandrill (*Papio sphinx*), each formed a new cluster of lentiviruses that fell more or less equidistant from the HIV-1 and HIV-2 clusters in the evolutionary tree. Neither was genetically close enough to HIV-1 to be a serious contender for the missing link. Crucially, they both lacked a tiny accessory gene called *vpu* (standing for viral protein U) that had so far only been found in HIV-1 genomes. Nevertheless, further research on SIV$_{agm}$ was relevant to an ongoing debate about the source and evolution of SIVs in primates and, by implication, HIV in humans.

The unresolved questions were basically how and when lentiviruses first infected primates. Two possible alternatives were being debated: the first was that the most recent common ancestor of all African Old World monkeys carried an ancestral lentivirus that then co-evolved with its hosts as they diverged into different species, a process that must have taken several million years. The second possibility was that a lentivirus infection originally restricted to a single simian species then spread by jumping from one to another. Either way all primate lentiviruses would be related to each other. Resolution of the controversy was felt to be possible by studying the viruses' individual positions in the lentivirus evolutionary tree. If they had co-evolved with their host species then the degree of virus relatedness would follow that of their individual hosts. On the other hand, if virus cross-transmission from one species to another had been the prime means of spread, then virus relatedness would perhaps mirror how close the ranges of these animals are to each other in the wild. However, as it turned out things were not quite as obvious as that.

African green monkeys are among the most common and widespread primates in Africa. They live in groups of up to eighty animals, each group occupying and defending its own particular territory. There are four different species of African green monkeys: vervet (*Chlorocebus pygerythrus*), grivet (*C. aethiops*), sabaeus (*C. sabaeus*), and tantalus (*C. tantalus*) monkeys that have non-overlapping ranges throughout sub-Saharan Africa. During the transatlantic slave trade in the 17th and 18th centuries African green monkeys were taken across the Atlantic as pets, and offspring of these animals now live in the wild on some of the Caribbean islands.

Well over half of adult wild African green monkeys in Africa carry a lentivirus in an apparently harmless infection, although the level of infection varies quite considerably between different groups. Many SIV_{agm} have been isolated from all four species, and in the evolutionary tree each clusters according to monkey species. Thus, although they are all related to each other, they are most closely related to the viruses isolated from the same monkey species even if the infected monkeys lived hundreds of miles apart.[1] This information, combined with the high level of infection in the wild and its non-pathogenic nature, suggests that these viruses have co-evolved with their hosts as they evolved from the African green monkey common ancestor several million years ago. However, other research provides evidence that SIV_{agm} has on occasions jumped to other species. Interestingly, and perhaps surprisingly, antibody testing of over a hundred African green monkeys from the Caribbean found no evidence of SIV infection. This suggests that the virus was only introduced to their relatives in Africa after the slave trade had ended, that is, in the last 200 years. On the face of it this seems to rule out co-evolution of the viruses and their hosts over millions of years. However, a counter-argument to this conclusion is that only young animals would have been selected for transport across the Atlantic: too young, therefore, to have been exposed to a virus that is mainly transmitted sexually.

Scientists looking for irrefutable evidence of cross-species transmission of SIVs have found SIV_{agm} infecting other monkey species including a captive-born, white-crowned mangabey infected with a SIV isolate from a vervet monkey. But as the mangabey must have picked the virus up from another species in captivity, probably through fights that drew blood, this only proves that under some circumstances spread to, and infection of, this species is possible. It does not show whether it actually happens in the wild. More relevant was the discovery of antibodies reactive with SIV_{agm} proteins in two free-ranging yellow baboons in Mikumi National Park, Tanzania, where the baboons live alongside a group of vervets. SIV_{agm} isolated from one of these baboons turned out to be a vervet-like SIV. Since the baboons in the park sometimes eat these small monkeys, this could have given the virus the chance to jump species.[2]

Another piece of evidence for cross-transmission between monkey species came from detailed examination of the genome of the SIV_{agm} strain in West African sabaeus monkeys. In the lentivirus evolutionary tree one half of its viral genome sequence clusters with other SIV_{agm} viruses, while the other half clusters with the mangabey and HIV-2 virus group. This means that it must be a recombinant virus which has arisen by SIV from a mangabey first jumping to a sabaeus monkey that was already (or later) infected with SIV_{agm} and then recombining with this virus to form a new virus strain. The evolutionary distance between the present-day SIV_{agm} strain from the West African sabaeus monkey and its two parents indicates that this represents an ancient recombination event between the predecessors of the modern SIVs in African green monkeys and mangabeys.[3]

In uncovering this microcosm of lentivirus evolution, these painstaking studies serve to emphasize its vast complexity. With evidence of co-evolution and multiple cross-species transmission events leading to virus recombination, the question of which predominates in lentivirus evolution remains unanswered.

* * *

Belgian scientist Martine Peeters was a colleague of Peter Piot at the Institute of Tropical Medicine in Antwerp working on STDs in the early 1980s when the first AIDS cases turned up at the clinic. The startling results of Piot's fact-finding visit to Kinshasa, Zaire, in 1983 (see chapter 2) stimulated Peeters to find out more, and in 1985 she got the chance to work on STDs at the Centre International de Recherches Medicales, Franceville, Gabon, West Africa. Here she and co-worker Eric Delaporte set up a laboratory to screen for HIV antibodies. However, as she found very little HIV infection in the Gabonese population she turned to screening non-human primates. She tested literally hundreds of primate blood samples for antibodies that reacted with HIV-1 and HIV-2 proteins. The samples were mostly from captive animals housed in the primate centre of the medical research centre where she was working plus a few from privately owned, household pets. Among her panel of primates were fifty wild-born chimpanzees (*Pan troglodytes*) captured in the tropical rainforest of Gabon. Just one of the fifty chimpanzees that Peeters tested turned out to have antibodies that reacted with HIV-1 proteins; a healthy, 4-year-old female chimpanzee that had been captured at the age of 6 months after hunters had killed her mother. While Peeters was busy isolating a virus from this animal, a second young chimpanzee was brought to the Institute in need of medical attention. Again its mother had been killed by hunters but this time the infant had also been shot and it had died of its injuries a week later. By a stroke of good fortune for Peeters, if not for the animal, this second chimpanzee also tested positive for antibodies to HIV-1. Peeters isolated a virus from the first chimpanzee and as she reported in a scientific paper in 1989, this proved to be a lentivirus that was related to, but not identical with, HIV-1. The amino acid sequence of the Env protein, usually the most variable part of the virus genome, was around 65 per cent identical to that of HIV-1.[4] In the lentivirus evolutionary tree the sequence of this new virus, called $SIV_{cpz\text{-}Gab\text{-}1}$ (for SIV from chimpanzee-Gabon-1), lined up as the closest relative to HIV-1 isolated so far. Significantly, it contained the tiny but all important *vpu* gene, until that time unique to HIV-1. Later scientists succeeded in amplifying part of the virus genome from the second chimpanzee's samples and this virus, called $SIV_{cpz\text{-}Gab\text{-}2}$, proved to be similar to HIV-1 and $SIV_{cpz\text{-}Gab\text{-}1}$, slotting into the same cluster in the evolutionary tree.

After four years in Gabon, Peeters and Delaporte returned to the Institute of Tropical Medicine in Antwerp in 1989 where they set about screening captive primates in Belgium for antibodies to lentiviruses. This screen produced one more HIV-1 antibody positive chimpanzee, an animal with an interesting history. Called Noah and 5 years old at the time of testing, he had been born in the tropical rainforest of the DRC (then Zaire) and caught as a young animal with the intent of selling him as a household pet. Then, when the animal was between 2 and 3 years old, he was taken to Belgium illegally and confiscated by customs officers in Brussels. The virus isolated from Noah was designated $SIV_{cpz\text{-}ant}$ (for SIV chimpanzee-Antwerp).[5] This virus also had a *vpu* gene, but, unexpectedly, when its gene sequence was analysed it proved to be quite divergent from $SIV_{cpz\text{-}Gab\text{-}1}$. Although its genome sequence still clustered with HIV-1 and $SIV_{cpz\text{-}Gab\text{-}1}$ in the evolutionary tree, it was twice as far from them as they were from each other, a distance more typical of SIVs from other primate species.

At this stage most experts thought that SIV_{cpz} would turn out to be the direct ancestor of HIV-1, but the diversity of the three viruses isolated and the very low level of natural infection (overall Peeters had found only three SIV-carrying, wild born chimpanzees among over 100 tested) cast doubt on this animal being the natural reservoir for the virus. As with African green monkeys, these reservations could potentially be explained by the geographical separation of chimpanzee groups leading to the accumulation of genetic differences in them and their viruses over time. It was also possible that levels of SIV infection varied between different geographical locations. Perhaps there were pockets of animals with high levels of infection in the wild, but with just three infected animals to study, two caught in Gabon and one somewhere in DRC, it was equally feasible that the viruses ancestral to those isolated by Peeters had jumped to both chimpanzees and humans from another as yet unidentified primate species.

This alternative scenario is not as unusual among viruses as it may sound; one recent occurrence being the outbreak of severe acute respiratory syndrome (SARS) that hit the headlines in 2003. The offending virus was tracked down to animals in wet markets in Guangdong province, China, where they are sold live for human consumption. SARS virus was isolated from several different animal species on sale in the markets, most often from the Himalayan masked palm civet cat which is farmed in the area. Indeed this animal was the likely source of the virus that jumped to market traders to spark the SARS virus outbreak, but the natural virus reservoir in the wild was later found to be horseshoe bats. With this in mind it was back to the drawing board for SIV researchers to continue the hunt for the missing link.

* * *

Meanwhile, across the Atlantic Ocean at the University of Alabama, Birmingham, US, Beatrice Hahn was also studying the evolutionary history of animal and human retroviruses, a subject that had fascinated her ever since she wrote her doctorate thesis on the topic during her medical training in Germany. She recalls that she was always more interested in medical research than in clinical practice, and so when she was offered the opportunity to train as a molecular biologist in Robert Gallo's laboratory at the National Cancer Institute in Bethesda, US, she seized it. Once there, she got busy cloning the genomes of HTLV-I and -II, the two retroviruses discovered by Gallo in the early 1980s. With her interest in virus diversity, she was certainly in the right place at the right time when HIV was discovered in 1983, and she undertook the genetic analysis of HIV in work that transcended any ongoing disputes over ownership of the virus itself (see introduction).

After three years in Gallo's laboratory, Hahn moved to the University of Alabama at Birmingham to head up her own research team. She began by isolating several new strains of HIV-2 from the Ivory Coast (see chapter 2), and it was as she was working on these and some SIV isolates that the big break came. It all began with a phone call from Larry Arthur, a friend and former colleague from the National Cancer Institute. As part of an HIV vaccine development programme at the Institute in the 1980s, Arthur had been one of a group of scientists looking for a suitable animal model for HIV infection. They had access to a colony of over ninety chimpanzees at the Primate Research Center in New Mexico where the animals were being used for research on hepatitis viruses. Arthur and colleagues tested blood from the chimpanzees for antibodies to HIV and came up with one sample that reacted strongly with HIV proteins in all of the five tests they used.[6]

The positive animal, called Marilyn, was pregnant at the time and soon gave birth to stillborn twins. She died a week later from a uterine infection and pneumonia. At autopsy enlarged lymph glands and spleen were noted, although the microscopic changes observed in these organs were reported as not typical of early AIDS. Marilyn had a long and complicated history, much of which remains a mystery to this day because somewhere along the line her records were destroyed when the building where they were stored burnt down. She was born in the rainforests of Africa, but her country of origin is unknown. In 1963 at the age of about 4 years she was caught and imported into the US. During her life in captivity she had fourteen pregnancies producing just six live young that were also housed at the Primate Research Center in New Mexico. Later HIV testing of these animals showed that she had not passed the virus to any of her offspring.

Marilyn herself was used in the US armed forces space research programme at Holloman Air Force Base in New Mexico in the early 1960s. It is unclear what part she played in this but she was later transferred to the primate centre where between 1966 and 1969 she participated in experiments on hepatitis viruses. As part of this research she received infusions of blood products, presumably from cases of hepatitis.

Arthur's phone call to Hahn was to offer her the remains of Marilyn that he had kept in his freezer for over ten years and was ready to discard. Since all other captive chimpanzees in the US had proved negative for HIV antibodies and Hahn had no access to animals in African primate centres, Arthur's call was like the answer to a prayer. She accepted the offer with enthusiasm, suggesting immediate shipment, and in early 1994 she received frozen samples of Marilyn's lymph glands and spleen that had been removed at autopsy. Arthur repeatedly warned Hahn to be careful—Marilyn had been infused with human blood products during the hepatitis experiments and so the samples could be contaminated with hepatitis viruses, HIV, or potentially something worse.

Hahn's research group skilfully amplified a complete lentivirus genome sequence from these samples. This sequence differed sufficiently from HIV-1 to be sure that it was not a human virus that had been transmitted to Marilyn via the infusions of blood products she had received. The new virus, called SIV_{cpz-us}, contained the critical *vpu* gene and was most similar in all aspects to $SIV_{cpz-Gab-1}$ and $SIV_{cpz-Gab-2}$, showing around 90 per cent identity in genome sequence. In contrast, the genome sequence of $SIV_{cpz-ant}$ was only 77 per cent identical to the other three chimpanzee viruses and so this virus remained an outlier. Indeed, the growing evolutionary tree now showed two distinct groups of HIV-1-related viruses, one containing the three similar viruses that clustered with HIV-1 isolates and the other represented only by the divergent $SIV_{cpz-ant}$ from Noah (Figure 8).

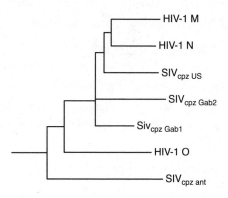

FIGURE 8 Evolutionary tree showing the relationship between HIV-1 groups M, N, O and the first four SIV_{cpz} isolates.

Source: Figure 4 in Sharp and Hahn in Cold Spring Harb. Perspect. Med. Cold Spring Harbor Laboratory Press. 2011.

Hahn had been puzzling over the evolutionary relationship between SIV_{cpz} and HIV-1 for some time when she had a enlightening conversation with her long-term collaborator, evolutionary biologist Paul Sharp from the University of Nottingham, UK. Ever since Sharp completed his postgraduate studies in genetics at the University of Edinburgh, UK, he has had a passion for analysing microbe gene sequences and teasing out their evolutionary history. So when the first HIV genome sequences became available in the 1980s he was ready to take up the challenge. He was the first to recognize recombination among HIV subtypes and is a key player in the ongoing debate over the ancient history of the SIVs. Sharp returned to the University of Edinburgh in 2007 via the Universities of Dublin and Nottingham where he had been analysing all the HIV and SIV sequences produced by Hahn's group for the past twenty years. On this particular day Sharp drew Hahn's attention to scientific papers on the evolution of chimpanzees published in 1994 and 1997.[7, 8] The information they contained was to revolutionize the group's studies and point the way to the final answer to the puzzle.

Remarkably for a primate species so closely related to ourselves, until the early 1990s almost nothing was known about the evolutionary history of the genus *Pan* comprising chimpanzees and bonobos (*Pan paniscus*, previously called the pygmy chimpanzee). The geographic ranges of these two species cover areas of the Cameroon and DRC, separated by the Congo River, with bonobos occupying a discrete area to the south of the river in DRC. Since both species are apparently poor, or at least reluctant, swimmers, the formation of the Congo River some 1–2 million years ago may have signalled their separation and isolation.

Chimpanzees are geographically more widespread than bonobos, occupying territories across equatorial Africa. Three subspecies with non-overlapping territories were recognized in the 1990s: the western masked or pale-faced (*P.t. verus*), the central black-faced (*P.t.troglodytes*), and the eastern long-haired (*P.t. schweinfurthii*). Although their names suggest that members of the different subspecies could be identified by their morphological features alone (coat markings and bone structure), in fact they could not. So since no chimpanzee fossils were available at the time, their definition was based entirely on their geographical location. Again, the chimpanzee's poor swimming ability was thought to have isolated the three groups, with the Niger River in Nigeria dividing the western from the central group, and the Ubangi River between DRC and the Republic of Congo separating the central and eastern groups.

Because of the difficulties involved in obtaining blood or tissue samples from these large and dangerous wild animals, genetic studies were lacking until 1994 when a team led by geneticists from the University of California, San Diego, US, began their research. They studied chimpanzees in Gombe, Tanzania's smallest National Park situated on the shores of Lake Tanganyika. It is here that the renowned Jane Goodall and co-workers have spent over fifty years studying chimpanzee behaviour and social structures. Goodall's research was by necessity non-invasive, and key to the success of this first genetic study was the development of a non-invasive technique for accessing DNA from the animals at Gombe.

Adult chimpanzees make new nests of twigs and leaves in the treetops every night where, except in the case of mothers and infants, they sleep alone and move on the following day. Ingeniously, the scientists collected hairs from abandoned nests and these provided DNA for their studies. The researchers obtained hair samples from forty-three animals from the Kasakela chimpanzee community in Gombe. This community had been studied since the 1960s and so individual members could all be identified on sight. Thus the DNA could be used for investigating social structures and historical gene flow as well as evolutionary relationships. For the latter the scientists also included hair samples collected from twenty-four animals at twenty other sites across the chimpanzees' range in Africa.

On the whole this genetic survey confirmed the morphological classification of chimpanzee subspecies in use at the time although it was clear that the western *P.t.verus* was genetically more distant from the central *P.t.troglodytes* and eastern *P.t. schweinfurthii* than they were from each other. Scientists estimated that *P.t.verus* must have been isolated from the other two subspecies for around 1.6 million years and suggested that perhaps it should be elevated to the rank of species in its own right. This chimpanzee classification was revised in 1997 when another group of scientists carried out a more extensive genetic analysis of chimpanzees in Nigeria, again based on DNA from nest hairs. They found two distinct chimpanzee groups in West Africa that differed from each other more than did *P.t. troglodytes* and *P.t. schweinfurthii* in the east. The most westerly of these was *P.t.verus* located in Senegal and Ghana, while the other occupied territory in Nigeria. Here they found that chimpanzees on both sides of the Niger River formed a single genetic group, now named *P. t. ellioti*. Their territories were still non-overlapping, but this research indicated that the Niger River did *not*, as previously supposed, act as a barrier between the Nigerian and central chimpanzees. Instead they suggested that the Sanaga River in Cameroon represented the divide between these two subspecies (Figure 9). Research is still ongoing into the precise classification of chimpanzee subspecies, but for the

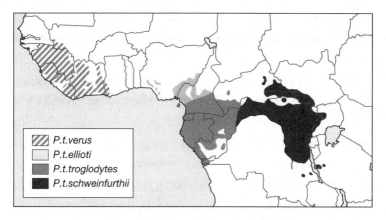

FIGURE 9 Map of west and central Africa showing the natural ranges of the four chimpanzee subspecies.

Source: Adapted from Keele BF, et al, *Science*, 313:523-526 (2006). Reprinted with permission from AAAS.

purposes of the work on SIV_{cpz} and its relationship to HIV-1 it was the definition of the four genetically distinct groups that was vital to unravelling HIV-1's direct ancestor.

On reading these research reports, Hahn knew that she must identify the subspecies of the chimpanzees from which the four known SIV_{cpz} had been isolated. This required blood cells from the four animals and since she only had access to Marilyn, she contacted Peeters in Montpellier suggesting a collaborative study. Peeters, who fortunately still had samples from all three chimpanzees (Noah, Gab 1 and 2) in her freezer, appreciated the importance of the study and agreed to send the material. Indeed, these two groups seem to collaborate and exchange this valuable research material in a gratifyingly collegiate and friendly manner, which has, undoubtedly, been instrumental in their success.

Instead of using chromosomal DNA, evolutionary studies sometimes use DNA from mitochondria, tiny but vital energy-generating particles in the cytoplasm of virtually all cells. Mitochondria are derived from bacteria that invaded primitive cells millions of years ago and to this day carry their own complement of DNA. Because mitochondrial DNA generally accumulates mutations more rapidly than chromosomal DNA it is ideal for tracking evolutionary relationships between individuals and subspecies. Using mitochondrial DNA from the four SIV-infected chimpanzees, Noah, Marilyn, and the two from Gabon, Hahn and co-workers found that three of them, that is Marilyn and Gab 1 and 2, belonged to subspecies *P.t. troglodytes* while the other, Noah, from DRC, belonged to subspecies *P.t. schweinfurthii*. On matching this information with the virus isolates all became clear; the three similar viruses, SIV_{cpz-us}, $SIV_{cpz-Gab-1}$, and $SIV_{cpz-Gab-2}$, came from *P.t. troglodytes*, whereas the divergent virus, $SIV_{cpz-ant}$, was from *P.t. schweinfurthii*. Thus the divergence of chimpanzee subspecies' DNA mirrored the divergence of the viruses they carried. The researchers concluded that, just like the SIV_{agm}, SIV_{cpz} had coevolved along with its host subspecies.[9]

By the time these results were published in 1999, HIV-1 groups N and O had been discovered in addition to the globally distributed HIV-1 group M. In the retrovirus evolutionary tree viruses from these three HIV-1 groups were interspersed by SIV_{cpz} isolates and were therefore not each other's closest relatives. This made it clear that M, N, and O viruses could not have evolved one from another after a single virus had transferred to humans. Thus, amazingly, the ancestor of each virus group must have made the jump from chimpanzees to humans independently.

In addition to this, all viruses in the three HIV-1 groups were more closely related to the SIVs from *P.t. troglodytes* than to $SIV_{cpz-ant}$ from *P.t. schweinfurthii*. This made sense in geographical terms as the territory of *P.t. troglodytes*, the central subspecies of chimpanzee, in south Cameroon, Gabon, and the Republic of Congo coincides with the location of HIV-1 group N and O infections that are mainly confined to the Cameroon. This body of evidence pointed the finger at *P.t. troglodytes,* as the natural host and long-term reservoir of the SIV ancestral strain to HIV-1.

Later studies monitoring the level of infection of *P.t.troglodytes* in the wild found, as predicted, that it varies according to geographic location but is generally higher than suggested by the early studies, even as high as 50 per cent in some groups. This discrepancy arose because the two other chimpanzee subspecies, *P.t.verus* and *P.t.ellioti,* are free of SIV$_{cpz}$ infection, yet the majority of the 1,000 or so captive chimpanzees tested in earlier studies were *P.t.verus,* thus giving a falsely low figure for the infection rate.

* * *

Construction of SIV lentivirus evolutionary trees involves scrutinizing sequences of virus genomes in minute detail, and this has revealed some fascinating facts about their history. For instance, the only fully sequenced example of the rare HIV-1 group N virus available at the time turned out to be a probable recombinant virus. More interesting though was the realization that HIV-1 was itself derived from a recombinant virus. Since SIVs are predominantly viruses of African monkeys, the fact that a similar virus should naturally infect the chimpanzee—an ape—was an anomaly that had continued to niggle. So where had the virus come from and how had it first infected chimpanzees?

As the hunt for more SIVs proceeded, the genome of each new lentivirus was carefully examined and located in the evolutionary tree. The number isolated increased from over twenty in the year 2000 to around forty by 2010, and the two that caught the attention of Sharp and his group were SIV$_{rcm}$ from the red-capped mangabey (*Cerococebus torquatus*) and SIV$_{gsn}$ from the charmingly named greater spot-nosed monkey (*Cercopithecus nictitans*), which does indeed have a large white spot on its nose. Analysis of the genomes of these two viruses revealed remarkable similarity to SIV$_{cpz}$, but only in certain parts of their genomes. Specifically, the *pol* gene in the first half of the genome from SIV$_{gsn}$ was most closely related to *pol* from SIV$_{cpz}$, whereas the *env* gene at the other end of the genome in SIV$_{rcm}$ resembled *env* in SIV$_{cpz}$. At first the explanation seemed to be that both monkey viruses were derived by recombination between SIV$_{cpz}$ and some other as yet unknown SIVs. Yet closer scrutiny provided another explanation—that SIV$_{cpz}$ itself was the recombinant. In fact the virus is made up from half of the SIV$_{gsn}$ genome and the other half of the SIV$_{rcm}$ genome. The all important *vpu* gene in SIV$_{cpz}$ and HIV-1 came from SIV$_{gsn}$ and is found only in this and a few other closely related viruses.[10] Today the territories of red-capped mangabeys and greater spot-nosed monkeys overlap with that of *P.t. troglodytes* in west central Africa, and since chimpanzees are known to prey on small monkey species, this provides a possible means of transfer for both viruses. Most probably either SIV$_{rcm}$ or SIV$_{gsn}$ or both viruses had spread to a certain extent among chimpanzees before they met in the single animal in which they recombined. Thus the ancestor of HIV-1 was born. Today both subspecies *P.t. troglodytes* and *P.t. schweinfurthii* carry the recombinant virus, so this momentous event must either have occurred before the split between the subspecies some 100,000 years ago or, less likely perhaps, it spread from one to the other since that time.

This meticulous series of investigations lasting over a decade identified the direct progenitor of HIV-1 in a particular subspecies of chimpanzee. However, as the scientists acknowledged in their published report, with only a few chimpanzees and their viruses available for study, there was still a chance that a monkey reservoir of this virus was lurking undetected in the rainforests of west central Africa. For this reason the team decided to study viruses carried by wild chimpanzees, but, as we will see in the next chapter, this was easier said than done.

4

From Rainforest to Research Laboratory

The groundbreaking work led by Hahn, Sharp, and Peeters identified a virus in chimpanzees of the subspecies *P.t. troglodytes* that seemed to be the direct ancestor of HIV-1. But with genome sequences from only three viruses to go on, all from captive chimpanzees, the group was hesitant in claiming that this animal was the reservoir of ancestral HIV-1 in the wild. Indeed a report from another research group in 2000 served to illustrate the problem. They identified three more HIV antibody-positive chimpanzees, Cam3, 4, and 5, all wild-born in Cameroon.[1] Cam3 and 4 were caught as young animals in 1992, Cam3 near the Cameroonian border with Gabon and Cam4 close to the Nigerian border. These two animals had been housed together, first as pets and later in a wildlife rescue centre in the Cameroon. Cam5 was captured as an infant in the central province of Cameroon in 1998 and transferred directly to the zoo in the capital city, Yaoundé. SIVs were isolated from all three animals including Cam4 although it belonged to the Nigerian subspecies *P.t.ellioti*. However, when the viral sequences were obtained from Cam3 and 4 they turned out to be ~96 per cent identical, indicating that the animals shared the same virus. Clearly one must have been infected from the other, and since Cam3 belonged to subspecies *P.t.troglodytes*, it was most likely that this animal had been infected prior to capture and its virus had jumped to Cam4 in captivity. Although long suspected, this was the first demonstration of SIV_{cpz} jumping between captive animals, so highlighting just how promiscuous these viruses can be. This underlined the danger of extrapolating findings from captive to wild animals.

SIVs obtained from Cam3, 4, and 5 were closely related to SIV_{cpz-us} (obtained from US chimpanzee Marilyn, captured in 1963) despite the thirty-year gap between their dates of acquisition. In the evolutionary tree all four SIVs clustered with HIV-1 group N, the very rare group of HIV-1 viruses found exclusively in the Cameroon. This at least showed that viruses similar to that isolated from captive chimpanzee Marilyn infected wild chimpanzees in the Cameroon, thus adding to the growing conviction that chimpanzees of the subspecies *P. t. troglodytes* were the reservoir of the virus ancestral to HIV-1. As always, unanswered questions remained: in particular, why were all these SIVs more similar to HIV-1 group N than group M and O viruses, when viruses from all three groups infected humans locally, with the pandemic strain, HIV-1 group M, being by far the most common?

Later, one more SIV-infected, wild-born chimpanzee was identified in the Cameroon, Cam13, bringing the total of known, naturally SIV infected, captive chimpanzees to seven. Clearly, the study of only seven SIVs from wild-born chimpanzees was too limited to rule out the possibility that a third as yet unidentified host for this virus might exist in the wild that had passed the virus to both chimpanzees and humans. For this reason Hahn and

Sharp determined to pursue the missing link in the chain to its logical conclusion by collecting and analysing SIV sequences from wild chimpanzees at different locations in the Cameroon and beyond.

*   *   *

There are plenty of reasons why research involving wild chimpanzees is problematic, particularly if the work requires taking biological samples from the animals. One obvious problem is that genuinely wild chimpanzees are exceedingly difficult to find. They live in communities of between 5 and 150 animals but their territories are in remote, often inaccessible, forested regions of equatorial Africa. Chimpanzees avoid human contact and although they are territorial they are constantly on the move, choosing a new nesting site every night. Even when a community is located the animals cannot be approached without extreme care since the adults are large and may be aggressive; mature males stand at around 1.7 metres and weigh up to 70 kilograms. Another problem is that numbers of wild chimpanzees of all sub-species have recently shown an alarming decline over their entire range such that they are now classified as an endangered species. One hundred years ago the chimpanzee count reached a few million, now perhaps as few as 150,000 remain in the wild. Also, when Jane Goodall began her work in 1960 there were about 150 chimpanzees in Gombe National Park, now around 100 remain. There are several reasons for this decline, not least the destruction of chimpanzee habitat. Over the past fifty years there has been massive, irreplaceable destruction of African rainforests as trees are harvested for timber or cut down to make way for farm land, oil-palm plantations, and human habitation. This has fragmented and isolated chimpanzee communities so that, for instance, the forest at Gombe, which used to merge with the surrounding forest, is now a 52 square kilometre forested island in an otherwise treeless landscape. Inevitably this means that chimpanzees are coming into closer contact with humans than ever before. As they are susceptible to some of the same infectious diseases as we are this has increased their death rate. They apparently suffer from flu and polio just as we do, as well as the highly infectious and lethal Ebola virus carried by fruit bats. After the outbreak of Ebola haemorrhagic fever in humans in Yambuku, DRC, in 1976, the disease was subsequently reported among chimpanzees in Tai National Park, Ivory Coast, in 1994. This outbreak killed a quarter of a 43-strong chimpanzee community (and, incidentally, jumped to a pathologist who performed an autopsy on an infected animal). Since then there have been several more outbreaks of Ebola haemorrhagic fever among chimpanzees, all with high death rates, and often subsequently spreading to humans via infected animal carcasses. According to a report in 2004, all human outbreaks of Ebola in Gabon and DRC in the previous three years began with someone, generally a hunter, handling the carcass of an infected animal—a chimpanzee, a gorilla, or an antelope.[2]

Excessive hunting is another reason why chimpanzee numbers are on the decline. Africans living in or around the rainforest have always used it as a sustainable larder but a recent rise in hunting poses a major threat to chimpanzee survival. Now hunters are not only looking for food: as villages and farm land encroach on the forest they also have to kill more often just to protect their families, dwellings, and crops from these large and destructive forest animals. But most worrying is the excessive hunting and illegal poaching of animals for the increasingly lucrative international trade in bush meat, now worth approximately two billion dollars a year. This deprives African forests of around a million metric tones of meat annually, and conservationists estimate that the market for bush meat is depleting the chimpanzee population by 5–7 per cent per year. Since female chimpanzees only produce one offspring every 5–6 years, the loss is more than can be replaced naturally. In response to this alarming situation the Jane Goodall Institute, the World Wildlife Fund, concerned governments, and other charities are working together with local villagers to address these issues, but still some conservationists predict that chimpanzees will be extinct in the wild by 2040.

* * *

The ideal material to use for virus studies is blood, but to obtain this from wild chimpanzees they have to be tranquillized with a drug-loaded dart. This can harm the animals, so clearly not an option given the present situation. Chimpanzee communities that live in parks such as Gombe National Park and Kibale National Park in Uganda are easier to access for research purposes as the animals are used to human contact. At Gombe they have participated in behavioural studies ever since Jane Goodall's revolutionary research began some fifty years ago. Her studies radically changed our thinking about our closest living relatives, and over the intervening years they have redefined our relationship with them. In general, chimpanzees are no longer regarded as suitable for experimentation, since they have feelings similar to our own that should be respected. Although important research continues into their complex social interactions, including interesting work aimed at understanding their means of communication and vocalization, today it is not ethical to use these or any other great ape for invasive research. Indeed, most countries have banned such studies on the basis that they can induce symptoms of anxiety and depression reminiscent of those experienced by traumatized humans. As a result, the world's population of captive chimpanzees has dwindled and many animals previously housed in research establishments are now in sanctuaries.

For all the above reasons Hahn and her colleagues knew that to have any chance of obtaining virus sequences from wild chimpanzees they would have to develop a non-invasive method of virus detection. Unfortunately the hair roots used previously to define chimpanzee subspecies contain host DNA but too little blood to yield virus genome sequences. So another source had to be found, and in reality there were only two options—urine or faeces. As chimpanzee urine was regularly collected by primatologists for their studies at Kibale and Gombe, Hahn managed to obtain stored samples from some of these animals.

The simplest test to set up was detection of antibodies that react with HIV-1 proteins, as it was already known to work well with urine from HIV-1 infected humans. Disappointingly though, the first batch of chimpanzee urine samples from Kibale gave completely negative results. However, when the second batch arrived, this time from Gombe, the group obtained their first positive result, proving that it was indeed possible to detect HIV-1 antibodies in the urine of SIV-infected wild chimpanzees. Compared to faecal samples, urine was more sensitive for antibody detection (detecting 100 per cent versus 65 per cent of infected animals), but when it came to PCR amplification of viral sequences, none could be detected in HIV-1 antibody-positive urine samples, whereas two-thirds of faecal samples gave positive results.[3] With this finding, plus the knowledge that it would be difficult if not impossible to collect urine from wild, forest-dwelling chimpanzees, the researchers decided that faeces were the best material to use.

It took two years' work to develop and refine the techniques for reliably detecting HIV-1 antibodies and amplifying virus sequences from spiked chimpanzee faeces. After this the team also developed ways of identifying the gender, species and subspecies of the chimpanzees. In the end they could even identify the individual chimpanzee that produced a particular faecal sample by genetic fingerprinting—PCR amplification of genome sequences that are unique to a specific animal. All these tests then had to be validated using faeces from captive and habituated animals of known SIV and HIV-1 status. With this done just one hurdle remained before they could begin their study on wild chimpanzees—the preservation of faecal samples between collection from the floor of the African rainforest and arrival at the research laboratories in France and the US.

Viral RNA molecules are fragile and are rapidly degraded in tissue samples by enzymes that chop up the nucleotide chain. The resulting RNA fragments are useless for genome sequencing purposes. Although this destructive process can be slowed by refrigeration and virtually halted altogether by freezing the samples, neither of these options is reliably available in the African rainforest. Fortunately, the team found a commercially available product that stabilizes and preserves RNA in tissue samples and this worked well with test faecal samples, even after subjecting them to the extreme temperatures experienced in the rainforest. With this in hand they were ready to go and, as luck would have it, Martine Peeters, now at the Institut de Recherche pour le Développment at the University of Montpellier, France, was working in Gabon and the Cameroon at the time. She was able to organize the collection of faecal samples from wild chimpanzee communities at various forest locations in the Cameroon.

In Cameroon, chimpanzees of the subspecies *P.t. ellioti* inhabit the area to the north of the Sanaga River while subspecies *P.t.troglodytes* live to the south. Chimpanzee communities at ten field sites were selected for the study, nine to the south and one to the north of the Sanaga River (Figure 10). Expert local trackers were employed to collect fresh faecal samples from the forest floor. In all, 599 were collected, each dropped into preserving fluid and subsequently transported to Peeters' and Hahn's laboratories. Here the scientists worked their magic to produce some stunning results. After the rigours of the journey, 513 faecal samples were sufficiently well preserved for successful RNA extraction. Sixty-seven turned out to be from gorillas rather than chimpanzees. This left 446 samples of the genuine article: 423 from *P.t.troglodytes* and 23 from *P.t. ellioti*. In line with the territorial distribution of the subspecies, all twenty-three of the latter specimens were collected at the site north of the River Sanaga. Antibody testing revealed that thirty-four of the specimens from *P.t. troglodytes* reacted with HIV-1 proteins whereas all the *P.t.ellioti* samples were negative. The thirty-four antibody-positive samples came from sixteen different chimpanzees, seven male and nine female, and viral RNA sequences were detected in one or more sample from each of these animals.

SIV_{cpz-} infected chimpanzees were present in five of the ten communities studied, indicating that the infection was geographically widespread in the Cameroon. Within a virus-carrying community the proportion of infected animals varied between 4 and 35 per cent, with the highest rates of infection in a site (labelled EK) in south central Cameroon and two sites (MB and LB) in the

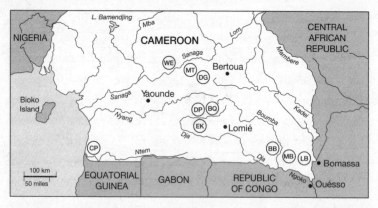

FIGURE 10 Map of Cameroon showing the location of field sites (WE, MT, DG, DP, BQ, EK, CP, BB, MB, and LB) used to study SIVs from wild chimpanzees.

Source: Adapted from Keele BF, et al, *Science*, 313:523-526 (2006). Reprinted with permission from AAAS.

south-east of the country close to the border with the Republic of Congo (see Figure 10).

All the viral sequences obtained from chimpanzee faecal samples were sent to Sharp for genome comparisons. The evolutionary tree he constructed revealed that the new sequences all clustered with the previously identified SIV_{cpz} from captive *P.t.troglodytes* chimpanzees as well as the isolates from wild-caught chimpanzees, Cam3, 4, 5, and 13. Interestingly, the cluster included HIV-1 group M and N viruses but excluded HIV-1 group O and SIV_{cpz} from chimpanzee subspecies *P.t.schweinfurthii*. This suggested that these two viruses did not originate from any of the collection sites in the Cameroon (Figure 11).

Detailed analysis of individual virus gene sequences provided tantalizing clues to the origin of HIV-1 groups M and N. The new viruses showed evolutionary-geographic clustering, meaning that viruses from chimpanzees in the same community were most

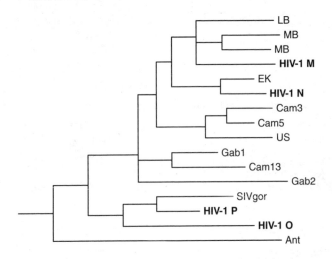

FIGURE 11 Evolutionary tree showing the relationship between SIV$_{cpz}$ isolates from field sites LB, MB and EK, from captive chimpanzees and HIV-1 groups M, N, O, and P.

Source: Figure 3 in Keele et al. *Science* 313: 523–526. 2006.

similar, and viruses from chimpanzees in communities that were close together were more similar than those that were far apart or separated by a barrier such as a river. This type of clustering allowed Sharp to pinpoint the ancestors of HIV-1 viruses to specific chimpanzee communities. HIV-1 group M virus sequences most resembled the sequences of SIV$_{cpz}$ from two collection sites (labelled MB and LB in Figure 11) in the extreme south-east of the Cameroon where one of the highest rates of SIV infection was recorded. In contrast, HIV-1 group N viruses were most closely related to SIV$_{cpz}$ from chimpanzee community EK in south central Cameroon. This was situated in the north section of the Dja Reserve within a bend in the Dja River, again a community with a high level of infection. The addition of these viruses to the evolutionary tree constructed from all SIV$_{cpz}$ and HIV-1 sequences certainly strengthened the link between these two lentiviruses. In their published report of the findings in 2006 the scientists concluded that:

> it is highly unlikely that other SIVcpzPtt strains exist that are significantly more closely related to HIV-1 groups M and N than the viruses from the MB/LB and EK communities [respectively]...Thus, an extensive set of molecular data all point to chimpanzees in southeastern and south central Cameroon as the source of HIV-1 groups M and N, respectively.[4]

This statement proved to be correct: to date no SIV_{cpz} that is closer to HIV-1 group M or N on the evolutionary tree has been isolated. Indeed, a later, more extensive study at fifteen sites in Cameroon confirmed the location of the SIV_{cpz} ancestral to HIV-1 M and showed that this virus was unique to chimpanzees in the extreme south-east of the Cameroon. Similarly, the SIV_{cpz} ancestral to HIV-1 N was again identified exclusively at the EK site; just across the Dja River chimpanzees carried quite a different SIV_{cpz} strain.

Publication of this remarkably precise location of the chimpanzee reservoir of ancestral HIV-1 group M and N viruses in 2006 drew a line under the debate over the origin and reservoir of the pandemic strain (M) of HIV-1. But the implication that SIV_{cpz} had jumped from chimpanzees to humans in these remote areas of the Cameroon on more than one occasion left open the possibility that other SIV strains capable of infecting humans exist in the wild. Having perfected the use of chimpanzee faeces to detect the viruses they carry, any primate species was now amenable to study, and scientists predicted that further surveys were likely to uncover, not only the ancestor of HIV-1 group O viruses, but perhaps also other as yet unknown viruses. How right they were, but even they were surprised by the next finding—an SIV in wild gorillas.

* * *

Gorillas are the largest living apes and are almost as closely related to us as chimpanzees, sharing a common ancestor with us around 9 million years ago. They are ground-dwelling, plant-eating, forest animals that live in equatorial Africa in troops of up to thirty animals. For all the same reasons as discussed for chimpanzees, gorillas are an endangered species. Their numbers are in severe decline and particularly distressing are several recent outbreaks of Ebola haemorrhagic fever among gorillas that have decimated whole troops.

There are two species of gorillas, the western gorilla (*Gorilla gorilla*) and the eastern gorilla (*Gorilla beringei*) which, like the chimpanzee species, have territories that are separated by river valleys. The western gorilla has two subspecies, the Cross River gorilla (*G. g. diehli*) and the western lowland gorilla (*G. g. gorilla*). The former's territory covers a small area in Nigeria and western Cameroon while the latter's range includes southern Cameroon, Gabon, Equatorial Guinea, and the Republic of Congo. The eastern species has a range covering an area to the north and east of the Congo River, and includes the mountain gorilla (*G. b. beringei*), Grauer's gorilla (*G. b. graueri*), and a possible third subspecies, the Bwindi gorilla (Figure 12).

Having, perhaps mistakenly, already collected several samples of gorilla faeces during the hunt for the chimpanzee reservoir of HIV-1, the scientists continued and extended their collection from the tropical forests of the Cameroon while also collecting samples from the as yet poorly studied Nigeria-Cameroonian chimpanzee subspecies, *P.t.ellioti*. As expected, none of fifty-five samples from *P.t. ellioti* contained antibodies reactive with HIV-1 proteins. But the shock came when 6 of the 213 faecal samples from wild gorillas turned out to be positive. These samples yielded three distinct viral sequences derived from three individual western lowland gorillas,

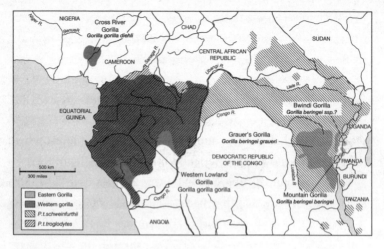

FIGURE 12 Map of west-central and east Africa showing the natural ranges of gorilla and chimpanzee subspecies.

Source: Figure 2 in Takehisa et al. *J Virol* 83: 1635–1648. 2009.

subspecies *G. g. gorilla*.[5] The viruses sat together in the evolutionary tree forming a unique lineage within the SIV/HIV-1 cluster. This virus is now called SIV_{gor} and is the closest relative to HIV-1 group O found so far (see Figure 11). Clearly this was a very significant find. Not surprisingly though, it raised many more questions, particularly regarding the origin and spread of the virus.

A more detailed evolutionary study on the gene sequences of the three complete SIV_{gor} genomes showed that the virus is most closely related to SIV_{cpz}, and just like all the HIV-1 groups of viruses, it is more similar to the SIV from subspecies *P.t.troglodytes* than that from *P.t schweinfurthii*. Thus SIV_{gor} must have arisen from SIV_{cpz} carried by *P.t.troglodytes* some time in the recent past.[6] The cross-species transmission could have occurred as a single jump with subsequent endemic spread within the gorilla population. Otherwise the virus may just occasionally jump from chimpanzee to gorilla in areas where the animals come into contact, without the necessity for onward spread. The finding of SIV_{gor} in gorillas living nearly 400 km apart, and the fact that the three gorilla viruses clustered together in the evolutionary tree, both tended to suggest a single introduction followed by spread through the population. To obtain formal proof of this, scientists screened viruses from chimpanzees and gorillas in an area of forest where their territories overlap. They found that the SIVs from the two species were quite distinct, having diverged from each other sufficiently to be sure that they had not jumped from chimpanzees to gorillas within the lifetime of the animals that carried them. This strongly suggested that all SIV_{gor} now in circulation are derived from a single virus that jumped from chimpanzee to gorilla, an event that probably took place in the Cameroon, Equatorial Guinea, or Gabon where the two animals' territories overlap. The estimated time of the jump is between 100 and 200 years ago, but this timing might be revised to an earlier date when more SIV_{gor} sequences have been studied.

Laboratory studies on the biological properties of SIV_{gor} show that it behaves in a very similar way to HIV-1 and SIV_{cpz}. It infects and replicates in CD4 T cells from both chimpanzees and humans, gaining access to the cells via CD4 receptor molecules in the same way as HIV-1 and SIV_{cpz}. Thus it seems reasonable to assume that the virus spreads by the same routes as HIV-1 and SIV_{cpz}, that is by blood and sexual contact. But exactly how gorillas first became infected with this virus remains a mystery. They are strictly herbivorous and therefore are not generally exposed to the blood of other animals. Nevertheless, gorillas have picked up other viruses from chimpanzees in the past, including hepatitis B virus that is spread by the same routes as HIV-1. Chimpanzees and gorillas often feed in the same areas of the forest and have even been seen in the same trees when these are laden with particularly enticing fruit. So it is possible that fights occasionally break out that are ferocious enough to draw blood, and that on one of these occasions the virus was transmitted. Alternatively, an indirect route of transmission such as contact with infected urine, faeces, or saliva could possibly have allowed the virus to jump species.

Once one animal was infected, the social structure of a gorilla troop provides ample opportunity for SIV_{cpz} to spread both within and between troops. A troop generally includes a dominant adult male, known as a silverback, a few non-dominant males, and several adult females with their offspring. The silverback mates with all adult females and so SIV_{cpz} would likely spread through sexual contact and perhaps additionally from mother to child. Also, young males leave the troop to live alone for a while before setting up their own troops and, when the territories of neighbouring troops overlap, both males and females may transfer from one troop to another, so providing the virus with the opportunity for onward spread.

At the present time SIV_{gor} is the closest known relative to HIV-1 group O viruses and, since SIV_{gor} arose from SIV_{cpz} relatively recently, a similar virus must exist in wild chimpanzees unless it has gone extinct in the mean time.

To date no closely related ancestral virus has been found in chimpanzees and so its exact transmission route to humans remains a mystery. There are three logical scenarios that explain the findings.[7] The first is that SIV_{cpz} jumped from chimpanzees to both humans and gorillas independently to become HIV-1 group O and SIV_{gor} respectively. The second possibility is that SIV_{cpz} jumped from chimpanzees to gorillas to become SIV_{gor} and then on from gorillas to humans to become HIV-1 group O. The third alternative is that SIV$_{cpz}$ jumped from chimpanzees to humans to become HIV-1 group O and then on to gorillas to become SIV$_{gor}$, although in reality wild gorillas are highly unlikely to have had contact with blood from an infected human. These different scenarios could be distinguished by the discovery of the ancestral viruses if and when more examples of SIV$_{cpz}$ and SIV$_{gor}$ are recovered and sequenced, as they would each slot into the evolutionary tree at a different place. For those readers who like brain teasers these are illustrated in Figures 13a, b, and c. If separate SIV$_{cpz}$ isolates are found that are ancestral to HIV-1 group O and to SIV$_{gor}$ then the first scenario is correct (Figure 13a). In contrast, if new SIV$_{gor}$ isolates are found that are ancestral to either HIV-1 group O or the whole SIV$_{gor}$ and HIV-1 group O cluster then the second scenario is correct (Figure 13b). For the third scenario to be correct then new HIV-1 isolates ancestral to SIV$_{gor}$ and HIV-1 group O viruses or the whole SIV$_{gor}$ and HIV-1 group O cluster would have to be identified (Figure 13c). The most likely geographical location for these discoveries is in regions where chimpanzees and gorillas coexist perhaps in Gabon, DRC,

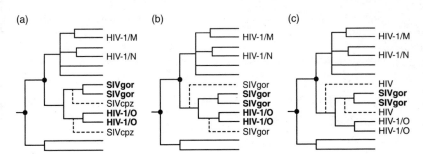

FIGURE 13a, b, c Evolutionary trees showing possible scenarios for the origin of HIV-1 group O.

Source: Figure 10 in Takehisa et al. *J Virol* 83: 1635–1648. 2009.

or Equatorial Guinea, but probably outside the areas of Cameroon that have already been extensively sampled.

The latest study tested samples from western lowland gorillas and eastern Grauer's gorillas but found SIV_{gor} only in the western species and restricted to sites in the Cameroon.[8] Even in Cameroon, just two of thirteen field sites yielded HIV-1 antibody-positive samples. This gave an overall prevalence of the virus in gorillas of 1.6 per cent, low compared to the prevalence of SIV_{cpz} in chimpanzees, which was 5.9 per cent in this particular study. The sequences of the new viruses isolated did not shed any further light on the origin of HIV-1 group O; however, there are many areas of gorilla territory yet to explore, so perhaps the key to the puzzle will be found lurking in one of these.

* * *

In 2004 a 62-year-old woman from Yaoundé, Cameroon, moved to Paris where she was diagnosed with HIV-1 infection. She had suffered from weight loss and recurrent feverish illnesses for over a year but did not have full-blown AIDS. French virologists were alerted when they found that her blood showed an unusual antibody reaction pattern against HIV-1 proteins. At first they suspected that she was infected with HIV-1 group O since this accounts for around 6 per cent of all HIV infections in the Cameroon. However, when they could not detect any group O viral sequences in the woman's blood it was clear that they had discovered a new type of HIV-1. A near-complete genome sequence was recovered from her blood that fitted into the evolutionary tree alongside SIV_{gor}. Because this sequence was more closely related to SIV_{gor} and SIV_{cpz} than other HIV-1 group isolates scientists knew that it must represent another transmission event. They named the new virus group HIV-1 group P (see Figure 11)—the fourth HIV-1 and twelfth SIV known to have jumped from primates to humans.[9]

The revelation of yet another group of HIV-1 viruses prompted a massive search among HIV-1 positive blood samples from Cameroonian donors for other HIV-I group P carriers. Screening of 1,736 samples revealed just one more positive, this one from a 54-year-old man in the Jamot Hospital in Yaoundé. No further clinical details were available but the virus sequence clustered close to the first HIV-1 P isolate to which it was 87 per cent identical.[10] Both isolates are even more similar to SIV_{gor} than are HIV-1 group O viruses whose closest relatives have been found in gorillas. Like HIV-1 group O viruses, group P viruses may have spread directly from chimpanzees to humans or indirectly via gorillas. Based on present genetic data the latter scenario seems most likely but too few SIV_{gor} sequences have been studied to be sure. So for now the mystery of the origin of both virus groups and the details of how and when they first infected humans remain unsolved. Further searching among the great apes of central Africa will probably eventually reveal the missing links—ancestral SIVs that provide the answers.

* * *

During the intensive search for the wild reservoir of HIV-1 group viruses little thought was given to the natural history of SIV_{cpz} in chimpanzees. Was it harmless or could it cause an AIDS-like illness in its natural host? Whatever the answer it was important to find out since lessons could be learnt either about immune mechanisms that impose long-term control over the virus or about its disease pathogenesis. This information could possibly lead to beneficial new treatments for HIV-1 infected humans.

The general assumption was that, like other SIVs infecting their natural hosts, SIV_{cpz} was non-pathogenic in chimpanzees. This is because SIVs are ancient parasites that have co-evolved with their hosts over millions of years, giving both partners the time to adapt to the other's presence. This was backed up by the observations that SIV-infected captive and wild chimpanzees did not seem to develop an illness similar to AIDS in humans or simian AIDS in captive macaques (see chapter 2). Even in the few recorded experimental HIV-1 infections of chimpanzees, AIDS did not generally occur. However, there were several reasons to doubt this perceived wisdom, not least because of the paucity of scientific information on which it was based.

At the time field studies on wild chimpanzee communities were extremely limited and those that had been carried out provided few scientific facts since chronic diseases like AIDS are difficult to identify either before or after death without laboratory back-up. Furthermore, a mere seven naturally SIV_{cpz} infected, captive chimpanzees, had been identified (Marilyn, Noah, Gab 1 and 2, Cam3, 5, 13), and some of these had died as infants shortly after capture. The only one that had been subjected to regular laboratory investigations was Noah who was still alive and well 25 years after capture (Figure 14).

Just two SIV infections had been studied in sufficient detail in their natural hosts to be sure that they were harmless. These were those carried by sooty mangabeys and African green monkeys. Yet there are substantial differences between these non-pathogenic SIVs and natural SIV_{cpz} infection in wild chimpanzees. First, the low prevalence of SIV_{cpz} compared to that of SIV_{smm} and SIV_{agm} in the wild and its uneven distribution among chimpanzee communities suggest that the virus may be a recent rather than an ancient infection. This proposal is corroborated by the fact that SIVs primarily infect African monkeys whereas chimpanzees are apes.

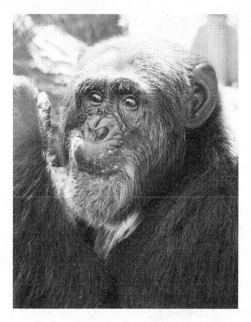

FIGURE 14 Noah; the first *P.t.schweinfurthii* with naturally acquired SIV$_{cpz}$ to be identified. © Mike Seres

Moreover the discovery that SIV$_{cpz}$ is a recombinant of two SIVs thought to have been acquired by a chimpanzee preying on their hosts (see chapter 3) suggests a fairly recent acquisition.

In 2009 Hahn, Sharp, and colleagues reported the results of a nine-year study on two chimpanzee communities in Gombe National Park. The Kasekela community, consisting of around sixty-five chimpanzees, has a territory in the centre of the park, while the Mitumba community which contains approximately twenty-five animals is situated to the north (Figure 15). Members of both communities are habituated to humans, having been studied continuously for at least thirty years. Over the nine years most chimpanzees in the two communities were tested annually

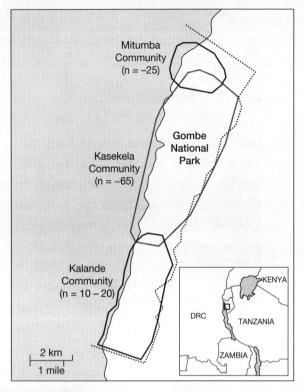

FIGURE 15 Map of Gombe National Park showing the approximate ranges of the Mitumba, Kasekela and Kalande chimpanzee communities. Inset – a map showing the location of Gombe National Park in Tanzania.

Source: Supplementary figure 1 in Keele et al. *Nature* 469: 515–520. 2009.

for SIV$_{cpz}$ infection by collecting urine or faecal samples. The proportion of SIV$_{cpz}$-infected animals in Kasekela and Mitumba was very similar, varying from 9 to 18 per cent during the study period. Nine chimpanzees were already infected when first tested and another eight acquired the infection during the study period. Two of the newly infected animals were infants of SIV$_{cpz}$- infected mothers and in each case the very close relatedness of viruses from mother and child pointed to direct transmission between the two. Four of the other six new infections were in Kasekela chimpanzees (two males, two females) who all became infected during a twenty-month period with viruses that were nearly identical. This suggested virus transmission between mating partners. Thus we can conclude that SIV_{cpz} is spread between chimpanzees in the same ways as the HIVs spread between humans.

The major new finding of the study came when field observations were analysed in relation to SIV_{cpz} infection. Over the nine years infected chimpanzees had a death rate ten to sixteen fold higher than non-infected animals. Furthermore, the birth rate in SIV_{cpz}-positive females was three times lower than in uninfected females and the mortality rate among their infants was significantly higher (reminiscent of poor captive Marilyn who had just six live offspring from fourteen pregnancies, see chapter 3).

Five chimpanzees that died during the study were subject to autopsy. One SIV_{cpz}- positive female who was profoundly weak and lethargic prior to her death was found to have multiple abdominal abscesses. In addition, her tissues were severely depleted of T lymphocytes—all very similar to HIV-1 infection in humans. The four other chimpanzees, two SIV_{cpz} positive and two uninfected, either died from old age or injuries. Comparison of their lymph glands revealed significantly fewer CD4 + T cells in the tissues of the infected animals. Taken together these findings demonstrate that SIV_{cpz} infection, far from being non-pathogenic in chimpanzees, causes a progressive immune deficiency that may result in a fatal AIDS-like illness. Moreover, the infection is detrimental to fertility and infant survival.[11]

Although SIV_{cpz} infection clearly has a negative impact on infected individuals in Gombe National Park the scientists were intrigued to discover exactly how much, if any, this had contributed to the overall decline in wild chimpanzee populations. To address this issue they compared their findings from the Kasekela and Mitumba communities with a non-habituated community of around sixteen chimpanzees at Kalande in the south of the park (see Figure 13). The number of animals in the Kalande community had been declining since 1999, due, it was thought, to a combination of illegal poaching and food shortage caused by habitat loss. Accurate monitoring of all three communities between 2002 and 2009 revealed that, while Kasekela and Mitumba were growing at an annual rate of 2.4 per cent and 1.9 per cent respectively, Kalande continued its decline at a rate of 7 per cent per annum. Virus testing then showed that SIV_{cpz} prevalence was around four times higher in Kalande than in Kasekela or Mitumba (46 per cent versus 12 per cent and 13 per cent respectively), placing SIV_{cpz} as the prime suspect for Kalande's declining population.

Scientists then compared the accumulated information on population size, habitat loss, chimpanzee mating, migration, SIV_{cpz} transmission, and death from the three sites. This was where the astonishingly detailed information they could extract from a faecal sample became invaluable. Alongside the observational data it provided confirmation of individual migrations, identified the fathers of young animals and revealed the donors of transmitted virus. All this information was incorporated into a mathematical model that provided simulations from which the scientists could predict the impact of SIV_{cpz} infection on the chimpanzee communities.[12]

The predicted level of infection that would result in negative growth and eventual extinction of the community was 3.4 per cent. This remarkably low figure indicated that all three Gombe communities were at risk of decline. However, the models demonstrated a fine balance between extinction of either the virus or the chimpanzee community that critically depended on the population structure within a particular community. Crucially, a community could be rescued from fatal decline by immigration of females from other communities, a process that occurs regularly at Gombe. Even if a proportion of these immigrants come from a virus-carrying community, the chimpanzees win the battle and the virus eventually becomes extinct. This is probably because, given the low level of infection in most communities, the advantage gained from new breeding females outweighs the negative effect of the virus.

With regard to the Kalande community, habitat loss was not found to be a significant factor in its decline, leaving their high infection rate as the most likely suspect. The death of four Kalande males in 2002, although not proved to be caused by SIV_{cpz}, was thought to be a defining factor, as it prompted the migration of several females and their offspring to neighbouring communities with no comparable immigration to maintain female numbers. Evolutionary analysis traced the origin of virtually all virus strains in Gombe to the Kalande community; thus, migrating females must have transmitted the virus from there to the Kasekela and Mitumba chimpanzees. Assuming that the lag period for SIV_{cpz} is equivalent to that of HIV-1 before clinical symptoms develop, that is nine years as estimated in nearby rural Uganda, the relatively recent introduction of virus along with immigration of several females has allowed these communities to continue to grow. But with the virus now spreading in their midst they and other wild chimpanzees have an uncertain future. Can a balance in favour of chimpanzee survival and virus extinction be maintained? Or will ongoing habitat destruction and isolation of chimpanzee communities prevent migration and tip the balance in favour of chimpanzee extinction? Only time will tell.

These models help to explain the patchy distribution of SIV_{cpz} in wild chimpanzee communities, and, interestingly, SIV_{cpz} screening of chimpanzees in several national parks only turned up infected animals in DRC. Animals tested in Uganda, Tanzania, and Rwanda were all negative. More recently, several communities of bonobos have also been screened for SIVs, and again all were negative.

The chimpanzees that have been studied so intensively at Gombe are all subspecies *P.t.schweinfurthii* rather than *P. t. troglodytes* that carry the ancestral HIV-1 virus. Thus we do not yet know if SIV_{cpz}-infected *P. t. troglodytes* might be similarly affected by an AIDS-like illness. Just one report suggests that this is the case— that of a male *P. t. troglodytes* chimpanzee (CAM 155) caught in 2003 in Southern Cameroon at the age of 1.5 years and kept in a sanctuary thereafter. He was SIV_{cpz} positive when tested shortly after capture and over the following nine years suffered recurrent infections and weight loss, with a declining CD4 count and high viral load.[13] This was clearly an AIDS-like illness in a wild-caught *P. t. troglodytes,* but field studies are warranted to confirm this conclusion in truly wild animals.

Having identified the natural reservoir of the predecessor of HIV-1 in *P. t. troglodytes,* in the next chapter we look at how scientists used the molecular clock to estimate the timing of HIV-1's jump from this animal to humans.

5

Timing the Jump

By scouring clinical records for the earliest AIDS cases and hunting through collections of frozen blood for HIV-1 positive samples, the traditional epidemiological studies of the 1980s pinpointed central Africa as the cradle of the pandemic. However, it was only after molecular virologists uncovered HIV-1's unprecedented genetic variability and defined its subtypes in the 1990s that Kinshasa, capital of Zaire, was identified as the probable epicentre of the pandemic. The mix of diverse HIV-1 subtypes and recombinants circulating in this city was unique; indeed, at this early stage of the investigation it was simply incredible. And when the oldest virus sequence in existence was amplified from the famous blood sample ZR59, taken in 1959 from a Bantu man living in Kinshasa,[1] the city became the focus of attention for scientists intent on timing HIV-1's jump from chimpanzees to humans.

Now it is important to find out exactly when the virus transferred to humans so that we can begin to trace its history. Epidemiological observations alone could take the story no further.

Finding answers to questions like how long HIV-1 had been in Africa, and when and by what route it spread globally, became the territory of evolutionary biologists. With their evolutionary trees, which, as we have seen in earlier chapters, are powerful tools for charting relatedness between individual viruses, they hoped to build a retrospective picture of the pandemic. At the time this was not just of academic interest. Having accurate information from the past could predict the virus's future evolutionary trajectory and thereby assist in defining a vaccine strategy.

We know that viruses leave no fossil records, yet the oldest HIV-1 genome sequences, like ZN59, are often referred to as 'fossil viruses' because they serve the same purpose as traditional fossils formed of solid rock. HIV-1's RNA genome mutates around a million times faster than the DNA genomes of other species, so although it has not been evolving in humans for long, the accumulated mutations are legion and can be used to track its history.

Once several HIV-1 sequences from viruses with known isolation dates were available it seemed quite straightforward to estimate the time to their most recent common ancestor using the molecular clock. To recap, the molecular clock assumes that the degree of genetic distance between two sequences of the same gene from different organisms, in this case viruses, is proportional to the time they have been diverging from each other. In an evolutionary tree this is represented by the length of the branches. So extrapolating back to the branch point, that is the point at which no differences exist, defines the time to their most recent common ancestor. On the face of it this may sound quite simple, but for the HIVs and SIVs, initially at least, it did not work according to plan.

First attempts to define the relationships between human and simian lentiviruses in the 1980s produced some wildly differing estimates. For instance, we now know that HIV-1, HIV-2, and SIV_{agm} are approximately equidistant from each other in the evolutionary tree, but in 1988 the date of the most recent common ancestor for HIV-1 and HIV-2 was estimated as 1951 by one group[2] at the same time as another suggested that all lentiviruses had co-evolved along with their respective hosts whose common ancestor existed some 25 million years ago.[3] Similarly, early estimates of the most recent common ancestor for HIV-1 subtypes were also somewhat variable. The first to appear was from Sharp's group in 1988. This was based on fifteen genome sequences from geographically diverse locations in Africa, the Americas, and Europe. It came up with a date for the most recent common ancestor around 1960.[4] This tallied with the report of the HIV-1 positive sample ZR59 dating from 1959 and was largely accepted for ten years or so. But when genome sequences were amplified from ZR59 in 1998, they provided new information that placed the virus near, but not actually at, the most recent common ancestor for subtypes B and D in the HIV-1 evolutionary tree. This suggested that the date of the most recent common ancestor for the whole of HIV-1 group M was somewhere between 1940 and the early 1950s. Another report published in the same year produced a date of 1942,[5] followed in 2000–2001 by three new estimates all agreeing on the 1930s.[6, 7, 8]

Some of the variability in early estimates for HIV-1 group M's most recent common ancestor was simply due to there being few sequences available in the 1980s. Also, those that were around had similar isolation dates, so giving a short time span for sequence divergence. All estimates used the molecular clock as

the basis of their calculations, which assumes a constant mutation rate over time, giving a linear relationship between the
number of mutations and evolutionary time. However, by the
late 1990s some began to doubt the validity of this approach, as
there were several theoretical reasons for mistrusting this basic
premise being relevant to SIVs and HIVs.

Although the molecular clock could only be used to investigate
the relatively short evolutionary life span of HIV-1 *because* of the
virus's high mutation rate, counter-intuitively, it was its rapidly
changing genome that was also the most obvious barrier to providing accurate estimates for the date of its most recent common
ancestor. The mutation rate varies considerably across the length
of the HIV-1 genome. Thus for the three major genes, *gag*, *pol*, and
env, the highest mutation rates, at around seven per thousand
nucleotides per year, are found in the most variable part of the *env*
gene, whereas the lowest, at around three per thousand nucleotides per year, occur in the most conserved parts of the genome
such as the *pol* gene. The reason for this is the variability in
immune selection pressure on different viral genes. *env* codes for
Env, the virus-binding protein that attaches to the CD4 receptor
on human T cells as a vital first step in infecting a cell. Antibodies
directed against Env block infection and so, not surprisingly, there
is enormous immune pressure for the selection of viruses with
mutated receptor binding proteins that are not blocked by these
host antibodies. But it does not take long for the immune system
to catch up and produce new antibodies that prevent the mutated
viruses from infecting cells. Thus, in an ongoing game of cat and
mouse, new mutants are selected. At the other extreme, the *pol*
gene codes for virus enzymes including reverse transcriptase, the
enzyme that converts viral RNA into DNA in an essential step in

the virus life cycle. Any change in this gene sequence is likely to render a virus non-viable, and so this region of the genome has a relatively low mutation rate. The parts of the genome with high mutation rates are called hypervariable regions, and in practice the region of *env* that codes for the virus receptor binding protein differs by up to 40 per cent between different HIV-1 subtypes, and even by as much as 15 per cent between viruses isolated from one infected person.

Given time, individual nucleotides in hypervariable regions may mutate more than once, and if this is not taken into account it would obviously lead to underestimation of the mutation rate. Furthermore, the mutation rate at different sites within a single gene may be different. In the 1980s the extent of these problems was not fully appreciated and so this at least partially accounts for inaccuracies of the early estimates of the most recent common ancestor. Evidently any estimate for HIV-1 depends critically on the gene sequences selected, so that in more recent calculations multiple, longer, and more represent-ative sections of the genome have been used. Also, the prob-ability of repeat mutations at a single nucleotide has been taken into account.

For dating ancient viruses it is often better to use the amino acid sequences of viral proteins rather than the genome sequences that code for them. These are more stable over time because not all nucleotide changes in DNA or RNA produce an equivalent change in amino acids. Thus they can be recognized and traced more readily. An ingenious study by Professor Mike Worobey from the University of Arizona, Tucson, US, and colleagues at Tulane National Primate Center, using lentiviruses from African primates on Bioko Island in Equatorial Guinea made this point quite clearly.[9] This island lies 32 km off the west coast of Africa and was cut off from the mainland around twelve thousand years ago when the sea level rose after the last ice age. The scientists obtained SIVs from Bioko primate bush meat specimens and found that each Bioko SIV had a counterpart SIV in mainland animals of the same species. The aim of the study was actually to resolve the controversy referred to in chapter 3 over when SIVs evolved, and for this these samples were ideal. Assuming that the island primate species along with their viruses had been separated from their mainland cousins since at least 10,000 BC, they used this date to calibrate the molecular clock. They then estimated the most recent common ancestor for a pair of viruses, SIV_{drl} and $SIV_{drl\text{-}Bioko}$, from the mainland and Bioko drill (Mandrillus leucophaeus poensis and Mandrillus leucophaeus leucophaeus) respectively. Comparing small RNA fragments recovered from these genomes produced an estimate of the most recent common ancestor for all the SIVs of around 49,129 years ago. In contrast, comparison of amino acid sequences of viral proteins gave a most recent common ancestor estimate of 76,800 years ago. Despite this discrepancy these results clearly show that SIVs are ancient infections. Of more relevance to the present discussion, the study demonstrates that the more rapidly evolving the sequence, the more biased the estimated date becomes. They concluded that calculation of the most recent common ancestor based on the molecular clock may be accurate for short time spans, perhaps for hundreds of years, but in deep time (thousands to millions of years) the accumulated repeat mutations can bias the estimates towards the present.

Before HIV-1 was discovered, virus recombination was a well-known feature of lentiviruses, and it was acknowledged that recombinant viruses could cause problems in evolutionary ana-lysis. The high rate of recombination among HIV-1 group M sub-types was first detected by Paul Sharp and colleagues right back in 1988 when they spotted one African HIV-1 isolate with an *env* gene sequence that clustered with other African isolates, but *gag* and *pol* genes that clustered with non-African isolates.[10] Yet this dramatic finding was virtually ignored at the time, the reason being that infection with more than one virus subtype, was con-sidered to be a very rare event. However, by 1995 thinking had changed. When Sharp's group reported at least 10 recombinants made up of two different group M subtypes among 100 viral sequences, it was accepted that these must have come from indi-viduals who had been infected with more than one virus subtype concurrently.[11] Once several recombinants were reported circu-lating in Kinshasa and other African cities, it became clear that dual infection was at least common enough to provide the virus with an opportunity to change much more rapidly than would be possible by single-site mutations alone.

Other problems that may have hindered accurate estimation of the most recent common ancestor for HIV-1 relate to the natural history of the virus in an infected person. For instance, the date of infection can rarely be pinpointed exactly since primary HIV-1 infection does not usually cause a distinctive illness. Researchers generally date isolates by the year of isolation, but given the long lag period between HIV-1 infection and the symptoms of AIDS developing, at this point the virus may have already been evolving in the host for several years. Alternatively, by chance the virus sampled may have been integrated into the host cell DNA as a provirus. This state can exist for many years during which the virus is effectively archived and not evolving.

We have seen how ongoing mutation driven by immune pressure within an individual produces a constantly changing population of viruses. One of these populations will expand and predominate for a while before being wiped out by the immune response and superseded by another. With viruses differing by up to 15 per cent in their hypervariable regions coexisting in a single person, sampling at just one time point may well not identify the predominant virus strain or, more importantly, the strain that is passed on to others. In addition, HIV-1's evolutionary rate varies with the stage of infection, being low in the primary and terminal phases when there is little immune pressure and high during the long lag period when the cat and mouse game is in full swing. Interestingly, sampled over the same period of time, viruses in people whose infection progresses rapidly to AIDS accumulate fewer mutations than those of slow progressors. Assuming that the rapid progressors have a weaker immune response, this again stresses the importance of immune pressure in selecting new mutants.[12]

These biological variations can cause estimates using the molecular clock to be somewhat erratic and so it was back to the drawing board for HIV-1 researchers trying to pinpoint the time of the most recent common ancestor for HIV-1 group M viruses. Over the years they have come up with increasingly sophisticated computer programmes that compensate for most of the identified variables. Referred to as 'the relaxed molecular clock', overall the revisions have had the effect of pushing the date of the most recent common ancestor further and further back in time. But before each new modification could be accepted it had to be validated on real live situations. Each group of researchers used sample ZR59 with its definitive isolation date of 1959 for calibrating the clock. They then attempted to reconstruct HIV-1 outbreaks from which several viral sequences from different time points were available.

One such is the well-documented HIV-1 epidemic that hit Thailand in the late 1980s.[13] With a population of 54 million at the time, the number of HIV-1 infected people in Thailand rose from almost zero in 1980 to 300,000 by 1990 and 800,000 by 1994. A snapshot testing of 600 people with high-risk behaviours in 1985 found only three positives, and a year later when, as a pre-requisite for obtaining work in the Middle East, many thousands of Thai workers were tested for HIV, all were negative. But by that time the virus was already in their midst. Having arrived in the northern provinces of Chiang Mai and Chiang Rai via the sex tourist trade, the virus entered the resident gay community around 1984. Then, with the government severely underplaying the developing crisis to protect the lucrative tourist trade, it spread rapidly. As is usual in a new epidemic, first hit were Thailand's estimated half million female commercial sex workers and from them it spread to their clients and thence to the general population. A previously unknown HIV-1 variant was isolated from the victims and named subtype E, but this was later found to be a recombinant virus and was renamed circulating recombinant form (or CRF) 01.

In 1988 HIV-1 began to spread through Thailand's 100,000 intravenous drug users, although on this occasion the focus was in Bangkok. This was clearly a separate introduction of HIV-1 since it was subtype B similar to that prevalent in the US and Europe. But it was the subtype E epidemic that interested evolutionary biologists. Because of its precise date of introduction in 1984, a date that was confirmed by the fact that genome sequences from viruses taken at the time showed very little genetic divergence, this was a good test for their refined prediction methods. In fact, the computer models came up with a date of 1986 for the most recent common ancestor of subgroup E viruses in Thailand, close enough to the date identified by traditional epidemiology to be very encouraging.[14]

Even more precise HIV-1 transmission dates came from a chain of HIV-1-infected heterosexuals that began in 1980 when a Swedish man picked up the virus during a visit to Haiti. He had eight subsequent sexual relationships, passing the virus on to six of his female partners. Two of these women later infected their male partners and two passed the virus on to their child. Thirteen years elapsed between the first and last transmission event in the chain; as the authors of the report point out, a time period equivalent to 13 million years of evolution in higher organisms.[15] After interviewing the people in the chain first hand, researchers defined each transmission date to within a few months, while stored blood samples provided viral genome sequences that had been evolving separately for up to twenty-five years. Using this information, scientists showed that the genetic distance between the sequences was directly related to the time intervals between their isolation, indicating that the concept of the molecular clock, albeit in a modified, or relaxed, form, finally fitted with HIV-1 evolution. Interestingly though, they noted that even at time zero, the branch point in the evolutionary tree, there was still some genetic distance between virus isolates, amounting to around 2 per cent in the hypervariable region of *env*. They concluded that this was because, as we have noted, each infected person contains a diverse virus population, so viruses transmitted on to different recipients will not even initially be identical.[16]

With a variety of modifications to the traditional molecular clock that allowed successful mimicking of these real-life scenarios, scientists then pinpointed HIV-1 group M's most recent common ancestor to sometime during the 1930s. But accurate calculations were still hampered by the existence of just one fossil virus, ZR59, prior to 1976 with which to calibrate the molecular clock, and this is where Mike Worobey came to the rescue.

Worobey is an evolutionary biologist originally from British Colombia, Canada, but his interest in viruses, and in HIV-1 in particular, began at the University of Oxford, UK, where he was a Rhodes Scholar in the late 1990s. As we shall see in the next chapter, he made a couple of trips to DRC to collect urine and faecal samples from wild chimpanzees and then teamed up with Hahn to study viruses from them, but relevant to this chapter is the detective work he undertook to uncover a human sample containing a second fossil HIV-1.

As an evolutionary biologist, Worobey knew the importance of archival samples for charting the course of the HIV-1 group M pandemic from its roots to its global dominance. And ever since hearing of the success of Ho and colleagues in extracting gene sequences from ZR59, he just knew that there must be more of the same out there somewhere. The obvious place to look was DRC. But several scientists had made the trip and come away empty handed: not because doctors and scientists in DRC had failed to store blood and tissue samples from the vital period in the 1930s, 1940s, and 1950s, but because during times of upheaval, especially the country's two civil wars in the late 1990s, all frozen samples had been lost in the frequent and prolonged power failures. Hence, the few valuable samples from

DRC that have been found, including ZR59, had been stored outside the country.

For these reasons Worobey first headed for Belgium, arguing that, as the colonial power in the Belgian Congo from 1884 to 1960, there must be Congolese samples stored there somewhere. The most likely place was the Institute of Tropical Medicine in Antwerp, and sure enough Worobey came away from there with a set of blood smears from Congolese patients. Presumably taken to diagnose common illnesses like malaria and anaemia, these consisted of just a thin smear of blood, perhaps from a finger prick, dried on a glass slide and then stored for decades at room temperature. Could T cell DNA and/or RNA possibly have remained intact under those conditions? And if so, would there be enough in a smear made from at most ten microlitres of blood to detect HIV-1 sequences? Luckily the PCR technique for amplifying genome sequences had moved on a long way since its invention in 1983, and after refining it still further Worobey eventually detected human DNA in the samples, but regrettably all were negative for HIV-1 sequences. Not deterred, Worobey then went hunting for specimens that would contain more genetic material than a blood film, that is preserved tissue samples. Every day hospital pathologists receive bits of tissue removed by surgeons for diagnostic purposes, and these specimens are first fixed, or preserved, usually in a solution of formalin, then embedded in wax to maintain the tissue structure. The block of wax containing the tissue is then cut into thin slices, which are placed on a glass slide, stained with dyes and observed under a microscope. Once the diagnosis is made, these blocks are meticulously stored and remain quite stable at room temperature for many years. As a daughter of a pathologist, I can verify that they never throw away their blocks or slides—I even inherited a set of them on the death of my father!

Until quite recently it was very difficult to amplify either DNA or RNA sequences from fixed pathological material, mainly because the formalin used to preserve the tissue architecture degrades DNA. However, there are now PCR protocols for recovering genome sequences from just such degraded material and, fortunately for HIV virologists, RNA is easier to access than DNA. With this in mind, Worobey made contact with Jean-Jaques Muyembe, a distinguished faculty member of the Department of Anatomy and Histopathology at the University of Kinshasa, and was given some tissue blocks dating from the late 1950s and early 1960s.

To summarize what must certainly have been a great deal of hard work over several years, just one out of hundreds of blocks gave a positive signal for HIV-1 RNA. But one was enough. Found in a lymph gland taken in 1960 from an adult female living in Leopoldville in the Belgian Congo (now Kinshasa in DRC), Worobey named the virus he extracted DRC60. To guard against reporting this exciting result only to find out later that it was caused by contamination with modern HIV-1 sequences, Worobey took the precaution of sending some of the valuable material to colleagues at another laboratory with expertise in HIV molecular biology. When they extracted the same ancient RNA genome sequences from the lymph gland material Worobey knew that at last he had genuine sequences from a second fossil HIV-1 group M virus from the so-called pre-AIDS era.[17]

In the evolutionary tree, DRC60 sits close to the ancestral branch point for HIV-1 group M subtype A. The genetic distance between this and ZR59, which sits near the root of subtypes D and B, is around 11 per cent (Figure 16). This figure far exceeds the genetic distance typically observed within an HIV-1 subtype, indicating that multiple subtypes had already evolved and diverged by 1960. Since a subtype represents several decades of independent evolution in the human population, this level of divergence implies that SIV_{cpz}'s jump from chimpanzees to humans to become the founder virus of the whole HIV-1 group M must have occurred quite a time before 1960. With both fossil viruses used to calibrate the molecular clock, Worobey calculated that the common ancestor of ZR59 and DR60, representing the most

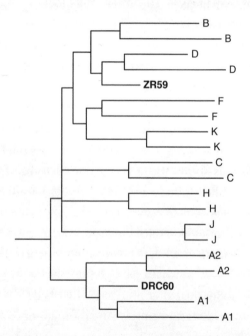

FIGURE 16 Evolutionary tree showing the relationship between HIV-1 'fossil' virus isolates ZR59 and DR60 and HIV-1 group M subtypes A-K.
Source: Figure 2 in Worobey et al. *Nature* 455: 661–665. 2008.

recent common ancestor for the whole of HIV-1 group M, fell somewhere between 1884 and 1924, and certainly no later than the 1930s.

Thus it appears that HIV-1 has been circulating in the African population since near the start of the 20th century. In the report of these findings in *Nature* Worobey speculated that the close coincidence of the date of the most recent common ancestor of HIV-1 group M and rise of the first cities in west central Africa (Kinshasa established in 1881, Brazzaville in 1883, Yaoundé in 1889, Bangui in 1899) may have allowed the region to become the epicentre of the pandemic. This discussion on the very early spread of the virus will be picked up again in chapter 7.

In line with what we know about the diversity of HIV-1 in Africa, in the HIV-1 evolutionary tree, both ZR59 and DR60 cluster with other isolates from the DRC, although, being older, they are both nearer the roots of their respective subtypes. Yet in the rest of the world, HIV-1 subtypes cluster geographically, with subtype B predominating in the US and Europe while C is the most common subtype in South Africa and on the Indian subcontinent. This shows that HIV-1 group M spread from Africa through so-called founder events, that is the seeding of single viruses which generated the specific subtypes in different regions around the world. How and when this dispersal out of Africa occurred was also uncovered by Worobey and his colleagues.

*   *   *   *

Back in the 1980s, just after AIDS was described for the first time in the US, the disease seemed to be more common in Haitian immigrants than in white Americans. In fact Haitians represented 5 per cent of early AIDS sufferers and for this reason they were briefly designated a high-risk group by the Centers for Disease

Control (CDC) in Atlanta, Georgia. Thus the 4H club was born (see introduction). This singled out homosexuals, haemophiliacs, heroin users, and Haitians, and long after CDC removed Haitians from the high-risk category the stigma remained.

Haiti with its capital city, Port-au-Prince, is situated in the western third of the island of Hispaniola in the Caribbean, the other two-thirds of the island being occupied by the Dominican Republic. In the 1970s Haiti was (and indeed still is) the poorest country in the western hemisphere. Malnutrition was commonplace and, as most of its six million inhabitants lived in appalling, overcrowded conditions without access to clean water or adequate medical facilities, infectious diseases were rife. TB, malaria, typhoid fever, viral diarrhoea, and sexually transmitted diseases all took their toll, and life expectancy was just 47 years. It is not surprising then that many of those with the means to do so emigrate to the US, and since Miami, Florida, at just 600 miles away is the closest point, this is where many of them congregated.

An early report published before HIV was discovered describes twenty Haitian patients with AIDS who were admitted to Jackson Memorial Hospital in Miami, between 1980 and 1982.[18] Aged between 22 and 43, and comprising seventeen men and three women, these people had all arrived in the US some time after 1975 and were therefore assumed to have acquired this mysterious, fatal disease while living in Haiti. The Haitians showed the typical symptoms of full blown AIDS—Kaposi's sarcoma as well as a catalogue of opportunistic infections, including *Pneumocystis* pneumonia, cryptococcal meningitis, thrush, TB, cytomegalovirus, central nervous system toxoplasmosis, and many more. All denied homosexual encounters and illicit drug use. None had immunodeficiency prior to their present illness but all now had low CD4 T cell counts. Half of the cases died during the two-year study, yet blood samples from some of the victims were frozen, stored, and then forgotten for over twenty years.

This report spawned wild speculation in the medical and lay press alike. With the revelation that HIV-1 originated in west central Africa still in the future, questions were posed about the role of Haiti in the origin of this puzzling illness. With insinuations about the significance of Haitian lifestyle circulating, the island's tourist industry died instantly. Everything from voodoo practices to promiscuity, drug abuse to dangerous health hazards came under scrutiny. Would a near-starvation diet combined with overwhelming childhood infections predispose to severe immunodeficiency? Could the voodoo practice of drinking fresh animal blood or perhaps blood-letting be a vital clue to the origin of AIDS? Had self-treatment with over-the-counter antibiotics or the recent swine flu epidemic in Haitian pigs spawned a new human plague?

When the dust settled, doctors from Haiti teamed up with a group at Cornell University Medical College, New York, US, to publish a report in the prestigious *New England Journal of Medicine* showing that AIDS sufferers in Port-au-Prince had the same risk behaviours as those in the US, that is, they were mainly young men who were homosexual or bisexual, had received blood or blood products, had frequented commercial sex workers and/or suffered from sexually transmitted diseases.[19] Unfortunately this did little to assuage the finger pointing and Haitians continued to feel vulnerable. The first authenticated AIDS cases in the US and Haiti occurred at around the same time, that is between 1978 and 1979, so the virus could either have spread from Haiti to the US or vice versa.

Since the 1970s Haiti had become an increasingly popular holiday destination for gay men. Fuelled by extreme poverty, Port-au-Prince grew into a hot spot of sex tourism particularly geared to the American gay market. A group of Haitian doctors argued strongly that the virus was seeded into the Haiti population from the US via this sex tourism. However, as researchers extended their evolutionary analyses to include the limited number of early Haitian viruses available, they found subtype B viruses that dated slightly earlier than the earliest American viruses. This hinted at the opposite scenario—spread of HIV-1 group M subtype B from Haiti to the US, but too few Haitian viruses were on hand to draw any firm conclusions.[20]

In 2008 Worobey managed to resurrect six of the forgotten blood samples from the Haitian AIDS sufferers studied at Jackson Memorial Hospital in Miami between 1980 and 1982. When he succeeded in recovering HIV-1 sequences from five of these samples he had the oldest fossil Haitian viruses in existence, a situation that he referred to as 'the next best thing to time travelling'. With these fossils in hand, Worobey tracked HIV-1 subtype B's epic journey from west central Africa to the Caribbean and in doing so made some remarkable discoveries.[21] As colleague Beatrice Hahn put it, 'It's a very nice piece of evolutionary sleuthing'.[22]

Worobey entered the new Haitian HIV-1 viral sequences into an evolutionary tree that already contained isolates from North and South America, the Caribbean, Europe, Africa, Asia, and Australia, as well as a few Haitian isolates from later time points. He then effectively asked his computer to decide whether the 'Haiti-first' or the 'US-first' model was the correct one. The computer did not hesitate. It unambiguously backed the Haiti-first scenario. Haitian isolates exhibited greater diversity than all of the rest of the world's subtype B isolates put together and were therefore basal to all other non-African subtype B viruses in the evolutionary tree. This pattern was similar to the unprecedented diversity of the whole HIV-1 group M in DRC. Thus HIV group M subtype B had unequivocally jumped from Africa to Haiti before it reached the US.

Worobey then went on to date the jump from Africa to Haiti by calculating the most recent common ancestor for all subgroup B viruses in Haiti. This turned out to be between 1962 and 1970, with a best estimate of 1966. Since all Haitian viruses evolved from a single virus, its entry into the country was the founder event from which all non-African subtype B viruses around the world subsequently evolved. In the next chapter we will revisit this date in an attempt to find out more about how the actual jump took place.

The HIV-1 group M epidemic in the US was likewise kick-started by a single founder virus jumping from Haiti, an event that Worobey dated between 1966 and 1972, his best estimate being 1969. If this date is correct, and most experts think it is, then HIV-1 was circulating in the US for nine years before the first HIV-1 positive blood samples were (retrospectively) identified and twelve years before AIDS was recognized. By 1978 around 5 per cent of sexually active gay men in San Francisco and New York were HIV-1 positive, suggesting that by then several thousands were infected. It seems incredible that the disease was not detected earlier, but perhaps the virus initially spread very slowly, with the epidemic only taking off when it entered a population of gay men with the highest risk lifestyles, and the disease only being noticed after ten years or so when symptoms of AIDS developed.

Worobey's evolutionary tree told him that the predominantly heterosexual HIV-1 epidemic in Trinidad and Tobago was also seeded from Haiti around 1973, again by a single founder event. This contradicted the previous assumption that the virus was introduced in the late 1970s or early 1980s through homosexual contact with gay men from the US.

The fact that single founder events carried HIV-1 from Africa to Haiti and on to the US and Trinidad and Tobago is not to suppose that only one HIV-1 group M virus made the leap to each of these destinations inside an infected person. Indeed, there is evidence that the virus, having used Haiti as a stepping stone, reached the US on several occasions and also jumped from Haiti to Brazil. But all these viruses, except one that succeeded in spreading to the US and one to Trinidad, produced dead-end infections that failed to ignite an epidemic in their new environment.

In general, founder events produce population bottlenecks, recognizable in a species' evolution by a sudden loss of genetic diversity as all future members of the species evolve from one or very few surviving organisms. Such a catastrophic event often results from adverse conditions such as lack of food or a change of climate. A common example is bacteria encountering an antibiotic drug to which they are sensitive. Virtually the whole population is wiped out, but a few carry a mutation that makes them resistant to the drug. These survive past the bottleneck and replenish the population with offspring bearing a 'fitter' complement of survival genes.

The spread of HIV-1 group M around the globe has been punctuated by a series of these bottlenecks and founder events that have caused the expansion of the multitude of virus subtypes we see today. With this in mind scientists have searched for evidence of selection of viruses with increased fitness among the subtypes, but have failed to find it. This lack of evidence for improved viral fitness fuelling HIV-1 group M's global spread leaves open questions of how and why the virus disseminated around the world. These are revisited in chapter 8, while in the next chapter we look at how and where the virus took its first steps in this global journey.

6

Vital First Steps

In solving the mystery of the origin of HIV-1 we have established *what* the AIDS agent is, *when* and *where* it first infected humans, *who* or *what* the virus derived from and *how* it spread. Now in the next two chapters we look at evidence for *how* the virus jumped from chimpanzees to humans and *why* it succeeded in spreading.

As soon as HIV-1 was discovered as the cause of AIDS in the early 1980s, theories about its origin abounded. But, excluding the outrageous, the incredible, the scientifically unsound, and the conspiracy theories, some of which are mentioned in chapter 2, what we are looking for is a feasible mechanism of virus transfer. This must assimilate all the facts about HIV-1 uncovered since its discovery and outlined in earlier chapters. By the year 2000 it was generally accepted that viruses ancestral to HIV-1 groups M, N, and O came from chimpanzees of the subspecies *P.t.troglodytes.* As these animals live exclusively in west central Africa, virus transfer is most likely to have occurred somewhere in this geographic region.

We shall probably never discover the exact circumstances of HIV-1's momentous leap, but since we know that the ancestors of each of the virus's main groups jumped from chimpanzees (and possibly gorillas) to humans independently, such inter-species transfer may be rare, but it is certainly not a unique event. We know that HIV-2 has made at least eight separate jumps from sooty mangabeys to humans, so these plus the four HIV-1 groups we have uncovered so far may represent just the tip of the iceberg. Perhaps SIVs have jumped to humans many times in the past but have either failed to take hold in their new host or were unable to establish a chain of infection. Either way, the virus would eventually have become extinct and the infection have remained unrecognized.

Inside their natural hosts, SIVs circulate in the blood and lodge in blood-rich organs such as the gut, lymph glands, spleen, and brain. These viruses are also present, albeit at a much lower level, in mucosal secretions like semen, breast milk, and possibly saliva, and so transmission between animals of the same species could occur through contact with one of these body fluids from an infected animal. However, since exposure to virus-containing mucosal secretions is a much less efficient route of virus transmission than direct exposure to infected blood or blood-rich organs, it is generally assumed that inter-species transmission such as ancestral HIV-1's successful jumps to their new human host were via contact with blood from SIV_{cpz}-carrying chimpanzees.

The most obvious human pursuit that involves regular contact with animal blood is hunting. In Africa, where modern man evolved around 100,000 years ago, our hominid ancestors have been hunting, killing, butchering, and eating animals for millions of years. Exactly when they developed the skill to make hunting tools of sufficient sophistication to allow large, non-human primates to be added to their diet is not entirely clear, although if the animals were old or sick they might provide easy prey. Today hunting for bush meat in those areas of west central Africa where chimpanzees have their territories is still a lifeline for many thousands of villagers who live in and around the tropical rainforests. Those of my colleagues who have joined villagers in their hunt for food testify to just what a bloody business it is to kill, skin, and butcher a wild animal as large and aggressive as a chimpanzee. They are in no doubt that the direct contact with chimpanzee blood and organs afforded by this process is quite sufficient to allow a blood-borne virus such as SIV_{cpz} to cross from hunted to hunter, particularly since bites and scratches inflicted by trapped animals and cuts from spears and knives are commonplace. But these observations are not proof and so the question remains: is this so-called 'cut-hunter theory' a true historical representation of events that took place around the beginning of the 20th century? Or did ancestral HIVs first infect the human race by some other means?

With no way of obtaining direct proof of the cut-hunter theory we are left weighing up the probability of this against other plausible hypotheses, some of which may be more amenable to testing. One such was proposed in a letter to the science journal *Nature* in 1990. This suggested that attempts to infect human volunteers with primate malaria could have provided the spark that kindled the HIV-1 group M pandemic.[1] According to the report, in 1922 two European doctors working in Freetown, Sierra Leone, tried to infect themselves with primate malaria by injection of fresh blood from a malaria-infected chimpanzee. It goes on to say that the medical literature records a total of thirty-four brave souls who were injected with blood from chimpanzees and a variety of other primates including mangabeys. The reasons behind these potentially fatal experiments, which would certainly not be given ethical approval today, appear to have been twofold. The first was to find out if primate malaria was caused by the same parasite as the human form of the disease, and the second to discover a better treatment for syphilis. At the time syphilis was a much-feared, incurable disease that was sometimes treated with a dose of malaria. This produced a high fever that was in some way therapeutic. Be that as it may, tests of this sort continued into the 1960s, the later experiments being mainly conducted in the US. The author of the Nature letter suggested that since both chimpanzees and mangabeys were used in the experiments, this might be a unifying theory for the transfer of both HIV-1 and HIV-2 to humans. Moreover, assuming that stored blood samples from the experiments in the US still existed, he thought that he had proposed a testable hypothesis.

This letter stimulated a response from an American doctor who had actually performed such experiments on prisoners in the Atlanta penitentiary in 1962. He maintained that direct injection of primate blood was never permitted by the local Ethical Board. Instead transfer of malaria was attempted via parasite-carrying mosquitoes.[2] Having admitted that no stored samples remained from the experiments he promptly dismissed the proposal on the basis that: 'It is a matter of scientific fact that AIDS cannot be transmitted by mosquitoes or other arthropods.'

During the 1990s the most seriously considered alternative to the cut-hunter theory was the 'OPV theory' of HIV transmission, meaning that the viruses were transmitted to humans via contaminated oral polio vaccine (OPV). This proposal first came to public attention in 1992 when a well-argued article entitled 'The Origin of AIDS: A startling new theory attempts to answer the question "was it an act of god or an act of man"' was published in the *Rolling Stone* magazine by investigative journalist Tom Curtis.[3] This American magazine, which has no links to the famous pop group of the same name, is advertised as a liberal, bimonthly publication that reports on music, politics, and popular culture. Curtis's investigation began in 1991 after he was contacted by AIDS treatment activist, Blaine Elswood from the University of California. Blaine had no medical or scientific background but is described by Curtis as a 'diligent sleuth of medical literature'. Apparently Elswood had picked up on the smattering of articles in the literature suggesting that HIV could have jumped species by way of a medical accident, specifically as a contaminant of one of the first live, oral polio vaccines ever tested in humans.

Traditional viral vaccines come in two forms: inactivated, where the virus is killed with a dose of formaldehyde, and attenuated, which contains weakened virus designed to infect and induce immunity but not to cause the full-blown disease. The first polio vaccine to reach the market was an inactivated product known as IPV (inactivated polio vaccine) or the 'Salk vaccine' named after Jonas Salk, the American scientist who headed the production team. Its distribution in the West from 1955 onwards caused an immediate, dramatic fall in the devastating childhood disease of paralytic polio. However, inactivated polio vaccine was deemed not suitable for use in the developing world as it had to be given by injection and required booster doses to induce life-long immunity. So the race was on to make an attenuated vaccine that could be given by mouth: that is, oral polio vaccine.

Vaccine production is a long and arduous process beginning with the growth of large amounts of virus in the laboratory and ending with safety and efficacy testing in experimental animals and then clinical trials. Viruses will only grow in living cells, and finding a type of cell that supported the growth of polio proved tricky. In the 1950s human cells were avoided because of a perceived risk of spreading cancer-causing genes, so cells from other animals were preferred. Monkey kidney cells seemed best at supporting the growth of polio virus, so these were used for production of all the early vaccines. At the time scientists knew little about monkey viruses, although in the 1930s Albert Sabin, the American scientist who eventually produced oral polio vaccine, isolated monkey Herpes B virus. This came from the brain of one of his colleagues who became paralysed and died shortly after being bitten by a laboratory monkey. Although this herpesvirus only causes cold-sore-like lesions in monkeys, it can be highly lethal to humans. Over the years several other researchers working with live monkeys or even just monkey kidney cells have died from its effects. Thankfully, a test was devised to detect the virus, and so we know that the kidney cells used for polio vaccine production, mostly from Asian rhesus and cynomologus monkeys, came from Herpes B virus negative animals. But the question is: what other viruses might have been lurking in the tissue culture mix?

Curtis's *Rolling Stone* article proposed that viable SIVs had contaminated some of the early trial batches of oral polio vaccine, and at the time this was certainly a plausible theory. As Curtis pointed out, a precedent for such a scenario existed in the form of simian virus (SV) 40. This, the 40th virus to be isolated from monkeys, was discovered in rhesus monkeys in the 1960s, a finding that immediately set alarm bells ringing with regard to the safety of polio vaccine. Retrospective testing of stored vaccine detected infectious SV40 in up to 30 per cent of both inactivated and oral polio vaccine batches. So even the formaldehyde used to kill polio virus in the inactive form was not sufficient to kill this new monkey virus. It eventually transpired that between 1955 and 1963, SV40 was unwittingly administered along with polio vaccine to around 90 million people in the US as well as countless millions around the globe. People given the contaminated vaccine developed antibodies to the virus, indicating that it had infected their cells. Worse news followed when SV40 was shown to produce tumours in experimental animals. Happily though, no firm evidence of harm caused by SV40 has yet emerged, although reports of tumours in recipients of the contaminated vaccine or their offspring continue to surface from time to time, so the case is not yet closed.

This cautionary tale served to illustrate that however much virologists of the day thought they knew about monkey viruses no one could guarantee that other, as yet unidentified viruses, were not hiding in the cultured kidney cells used to grow polio virus for vaccine production. Indeed, in the 1950s virologists were completely unaware of the existence of SIVs which, as latent viruses, can infect cells for a lifetime without showing any outward signs of their presence. However, following this scare and a ban on the export of rhesus monkeys by the Indian government in the 1950s (which was just a temporary ban but no one knew that at the time), scientists switched to using kidneys from African green monkeys. We now know that SIV_{agm} is only distantly related to the HIVs, but it was SIV from these animals that Curtis identified in his article as the possible ancestor of HIV.

The oral polio vaccine that was eventually approved for use was produced by Sabin in the 1960s, but prior to this there was immense competition between research groups for this lucrative prize. One competitor, Hilary Koprowski, developed an oral polio vaccine at the Wistar Institute, Philadelphia, US, where he was the Director. Koprowski produced an early, experimental vaccine called CHAT that was the first oral polio vaccine ever to be used in mass vaccination trials. Initially it was tested in a small number of institutionalized, mentally handicapped children and the infants of women prisoners in the US. It was also used in several European countries, but the first large-scale trials were in Africa. The vaccination team reported this mass polio vaccination campaign in the *British Medical Journal* in 1958, stating that CHAT had been administered via an oral spray to 244,596 inhabitants of the Belgian Congo and Ruanda-Urundi.[4] The largest programme was in the Ruzizi Valley bordering on today's DRC, Rwanda, and Burundi in central Africa. After being directed to assemble at a prearranged rallying point by their village chiefs, three to ten thousand people queued and were vaccinated daily between February and April 1957. In all 215,504 people in the valley received the oral vaccine. Then, as a polio epidemic swept through the region, further campaigns were undertaken in affected towns and villages including the capital, Leopoldville (now Kinshasa). By the end of the campaign around a million people in the area had been vaccinated, most of whom were young children.

In the *Rolling Stone* article Curtis noted that the site of these vaccination campaigns coincided with the geographic areas where some of the highest levels of HIV-1 infection and the earliest AIDS cases occurred around twenty years later. Also the timing of the campaigns fitted neatly with the date of 1960 proposed for the most recent common ancestor of HIV-1 group M viruses by evolutionary biologists at the time (see chapter 5).[5] Consequently, Curtis pointed the finger at these African field trials as the possible origin of the HIV-1 pandemic. Indeed, he suggested that SIV_{agm} had contaminated the vaccine, infected vaccine recipients, and evolved into HIV-1. As a result, Koprowski sued Curtis and the *Rolling Stone* magazine for defamation. The case was eventually settled out of court, with the magazine editors agreeing to publish a 'clarification note' stating that Dr Koprowski was an illustrious scientist and that in the article they had not intended to suggest that there was any scientific proof that he was responsible for introducing AIDS to the human population. They were ordered to pay Koprowski the sum of $1 in damages while their legal fees amounted to half a million dollars.[6]

Not surprisingly, following this event Curtis was discouraged from publishing on the polio vaccine/AIDS story. However, a British writer and journalist, Edward Hooper, emerged to assume the role of champion for the theory. Over the next few years he carried out painstaking research into the background of the allegations implicit in the theory. He travelled around the globe, interviewed more than 600 people involved in vaccine production and testing, prised out the unpublished minutiae of laboratory protocols and procedures and uncovered some rather unconventional practices. When it became obvious that SIV_{agm} is only distantly related to HIV-1 he suggested that the vaccine virus may have been grown in chimpanzee kidney cells, and hence SIV_{cpz} could have been transmitted to humans. In 1999 he published *The River: A journey to the source of HIV and AIDS,*[7] an extraordinary book of over 1,000 pages with close to 2,500 footnotes, that details the history of every facet of the HIV/AIDS pandemic. This encompassed not only HIV-1 group M but also groups N and O and HIV-2, all of which Hooper now included in the oral polio vaccine theory.

By the end of his investigation Hooper believed that some scientists, researchers, journal editors, and doctors had colluded to prevent exposure of a possible medical mishap as the cause the devastating HIV pandemic. One very eminent scientist was open minded enough to take up the cause. This was William (Bill) Hamilton, Royal Society Professor of Evolutionary Biology at the University of Oxford, UK, who wrote in the forward to *The River*: 'The thesis in The River is that the closing of the ranks against inquiry may, in this case, be preventing proper discussion of an accident that is bidding to prove itself more expensive in lives than all human attritions put in motion by Hitler, Stalin and Pol Pot.'[8]

In truth, a minority of scientists and doctors *were* unwilling to entertain the possibility that their vaccine could have been at the root of the devastating pandemic. Unsurprisingly this included those directly involved in oral polio vaccine production and testing, who, after all, had been acting in good faith to save thousands of lives. Others felt strongly that since nothing could be done to reverse past events it was better to leave well alone because the oral polio vaccine theory, if true, would destroy the public's faith in vaccination. However, most thought it worth investigating, considering that it was important to uncover the facts so that, if the theory was true, such a tragedy could be avoided in the future. As originally suggested by Curtis, an expert committee was set up by the Wistar Institute to investigate the theory. In 1992 it pronounced: '... we consider the probability of the AIDs epidemic having been started by the inadvertent inoculation of an unknown HIV precursor into African children during the 1957 poliovirus vaccine trials to be extremely low. Almost every step in this hypothetical mode of transmission is problematic.'[9]

Probably most HIV experts agreed with this conclusion, but no one could categorically state that early batches of CHAT had not contained SIVs. In the production line SIV-carrying immune cells *could* have contaminated monkey kidney cell cultures if the kidney donors were SIV infected. SIVs *could* have survived the vaccine preparation process because no virus inactivation step was included. SIVs *could* have infected vaccinees via the oral spray since HIV can infect by the oral route. The infectivity of SIVs *could* have been enhanced by the young age of most vaccinees and the possible presence of mouth sores, wounds, or blisters. Furthermore, the vaccine spray *could* have reached the respiratory tract where there are cells that are certainly susceptible to HIV infection. The fact that no AIDS cases resulted from the CHAT trials outside Africa *could* be explained if only a few vaccine batches were SIV contaminated.

The expert committee cited the case of the Manchester sailor who developed AIDS-like symptoms in the UK in 1958 as evidence against the oral polio vaccine theory since this was too early to be related to the CHAT trials. However, as we saw in chapter 2, by 1995 it was clear that this case of immunodeficiency was unrelated to HIV infection.[10] They also mention the first known HIV-1 antibody positive blood sample, ZR59, taken in Leopoldville in 1959. Timewise this could have come from someone who had just received polio vaccine in the Leopoldville trial which was going on around that time. But although the ZR59 virus had not yet been sequenced, the committee pointed out that the evolutionary distance between any known SIVs and HIV-1 could not be bridged in such a short time.

Hamilton was particularly struck by the remarkable coincidence of the polio vaccine trials and early evidence of HIV infection and AIDS in the Ruzizi Valley. So, although he did not necessarily believe the theory, he felt strongly that it deserved serious consideration by the scientific community. In pushing for its recognition he persuaded the Royal Society in London to hold a discussion meeting at which the subject could be aired and debated. This finally came about in 2000, but in the meantime Hamilton was keen to help establish some facts. He identified the two key lines of investigation as, first, to ascertain whether chimpanzee kidneys had ever been used in the production of CHAT and if so whether the animals carried an SIV closely related to HIV-1; second, to find out if any stored batches of CHAT still existed and test them for SIVs as well as cellular DNA. The latter test would identify the origin of the primate cells used to grow the vaccine virus. Both of these tasks proved more difficult than expected.

Koprowski maintained that only rhesus monkey kidneys from India and the Philippines had been used for production of CHAT vaccine but he could provide few laboratory records to verify this. It seems that kidneys were sometimes removed from animals before transport to the US, so that laboratory workers were not always aware of which species they came from. Hooper postulated that when the cut in kidney supply line from Asia threatened to cause a severe shortage, organs from a variety of primate species from Africa may have been used. This possibly included chimpanzee kidneys since these animals were already used for vaccine safety and efficacy testing.[11]

For the CHAT vaccine used in the African trials these tests were carried out at an experimental research station, Camp Lindi, situated in the rainforest near Stanleyville (now Kisangani) in the north-east of the Belgian Congo. This facility opened specifically for polio vaccine testing as a prelude to the large trials planned in the area. The research station housed chimpanzees and bonobos that were caught in the surrounding Parisi Forest by local hunters.

The animals either received intra-spinal injections of vaccine to ascertain that it was harmless or they were given oral polio vaccine and then challenged with wild polio virus to ensure that the vaccine induced immunity.

Hamilton and Hooper visited Kisangani in 1999, Hooper to investigate the goings on at Camp Lindi, which by that time had long since shut down, and Hamilton to try to locate a population of chimpanzees that carried SIVs ancestral to HIV-1. According to Hooper: 'Camp Lindi opened in June 1956.... by February 1958, 20 months later, the number of chimps that had been present at Lindi had reached 416'.[12] But by the end of the polio trials most had been sacrificed; only around fifty animals remained. So Hooper's question was: what happened to the organs from the animals that had been killed? Detailed records were either missing or incomplete but he became convinced that on occasions chimpanzee kidneys were used to grow virus in the final stages of CHAT vaccine preparation, either locally or after being sent to Koprowski's laboratory in the US.[13]

On his first visit to Kisangani Hamilton was only able to obtain samples from pet chimpanzees and no viruses survived the journey home, but as Hooper's suspicions grew so did the need to investigate viruses carried by local wild chimpanzees. So in early 2000 Hamilton visited Kisangani again, this time accompanied by evolutionary biologist Mike Worobey who was then at the University of Oxford, UK. Although sceptical about the oral polio vaccine theory, Worobey was keen to obtain SIVs from wild chimpanzees in DRC for evolutionary studies. This time they succeeded in collecting both faeces and urine from wild *P.t schweinfurthii* chimpanzees local to the area that later yielded SIVs. But this success was overshadowed by the fateful outcome of the trip.

Led by local guides, they were two days into the forest when Worobey impaled his hand on an overhanging spiny branch that left an inch-long splinter imbedded in his thumb. With no antibiotics available the wound became infected, turned black and in no time at all Worobey was seriously unwell. Luckily he made it out of the forest clutching the first chimpanzee samples they had collected. With the splinter removed and the appropriate antibiotics provided by the independent medical aid organization, Médecins Sans Frontières, he made a full recovery. But much worse was to follow. With the rainforest mission complete and everyone back in Kisangani, in self-congratulatory mood, Hamilton unexpectedly woke the next morning with the high fever, profuse sweating, and chills of malaria. There followed a nightmarish dash to the airport for the first available flight out. This took them to Kampala in Uganda where Hamilton got anti-malarial treatment. They then travelled rapidly on to London via Nairobi and by the time they touched down at Heathrow the parasite was apparently vanquished from his system. Sadly though, Hamilton collapsed the next day and died three weeks later. He was 63 years old.

I never met Hamilton and was only introduced to his work through its popularization by Richard Dawkins in *The Selfish Gene*.[14] What shines through from the many published obituaries is how much Hamilton was loved and respected by friends, colleagues, and students alike, both for his unique form of genius and his unconventionality. The following quotes give a flavour of the man: he was 'a gentle giant', 'a solitary scholar', 'a one-off', with 'a radical originality' and 'a distain for authority'.[15, 16, 17]

Despite Hamilton's death in March 2000, the discussion meeting hosted by the Royal Society that he had instigated went ahead in London later the same year. Feelings were running high, and controversy over the list of invited speakers generated heated debate in the press, causing the meeting to be postponed. In the end it took place in September 2000, with all the main players assembled to present their evidence and discuss the pros and cons of the oral polio vaccine and other theories of how the HIVs jumped from primates to humans. Contributors included experts in virology, polio virus vaccine, epidemiology, molecular and evolutionary biology, and the oral polio vaccine theory. Clearly this was an explosive mix and Worobey recalls a scientific meeting with 'a uniquely adversarial tone to the discussions'.

Many issues were debated at the meeting, the proceedings of which were later published.[18] The main points were these:

- In the early 1990s when Curtis first published the theory of the origin of HIV-1 in humans and Hooper, later joined by Hamilton, began seeking evidence to support it, evolutionary biologists placed the date of the most recent common ancestor for HIV-1 group M at around 1960. However, as discussed in chapter 5, during the intervening years these same scientists, having refined their techniques and accumulated more virus sequences, revised this estimate to an earlier date. By the time of the Royal Society meeting there was general consensus that the date of the most recent common ancestor for HIV-1 group M was between 1915 and 1941, the best estimate being 1931. This was obviously too early for contaminated polio vaccine to be blamed for its transfer to humans. Since the date itself gives no clues as to the host species in which the most recent common ancestor resided, Hooper produced a counterargument. He accepted that HIV-1 group M could have evolved in the 1930s but suggested (without any supporting evidence) that this occurred in chimpanzees rather than humans. He postulated that the virus had diversified into its ten or so subtypes in chimpanzees, each of which was then transmitted to humans via oral polio vaccine in the late 1950s. He went on to propose that the very distinctive 'starburst' structure in the HIV-1 M evolutionary tree, caused by the almost simultaneous evolution of the subgroups, is best explained by their transfer via contaminated vaccine over the two-year period of the vaccination campaign in the Ruzizi Valley.

- At the time of the meeting in 2000, the studies by Hahn, Sharp, and Peeters that found ancestral HIV-1 group M in wild *P.t. troglodytes* chimpanzees in south-east Cameroon (see chapter 4) had not been reported. Thus the assumption that *P.t. troglodytes* was the source of this virus in humans was based on just seven SIV_{cpz} isolates from captive animals and the identity of the natural reservoir of this virus was still uncertain. Nevertheless it was clear that Camp Lindi, situated in the north-east of DRC, was within the range of the eastern chimpanzee subspecies *P.t.schweinfurthii* rather than the central subspecies, *P.t. troglodytes*. On this basis Sharp argued that the chimpanzees at Camp Lindi that Hooper believed had been used to make kidney cell cultures did not carry the SIV ancestral to HIV-1 group M. In any case, as expected, the scientists directly involved in CHAT vaccine production denied that chimpanzee kidneys were ever used for polio virus propagation at any of the production sites in the US or Europe. Furthermore, neither polio virus propagation nor vaccine production could have taken place at Camp Lindi since the research station did not possess a tissue culture facility suitable for such procedures.

- In their 1992 report on the oral polio vaccine theory the AIDS/ Poliovirus Advisory Committee to the Wistar Institute had declared that 'some testing of available [stored vaccine] samples may be desirable so that no stone is left unturned'.[19] This testing was to look for evidence of HIV or SIV contamination of batches of CHAT vaccine, and in 1999 Hamilton had additionally advocated testing the material for host cell DNA to identify the species of the cells in which the virus had been grown. This proved to be a long and complicated process with several experts refusing to get involved. Despite this, the results of tests carried out at the Wistar Institute and other independent laboratories were finally ready for presentation at the meeting. All the vaccine batches tested proved negative for primate lentivirus sequences. In those in which host genome sequences could be detected, the origin of the cultured cells was identified as Asian macaques and not chimpanzees. Thus this provided no evidence to support the oral polio vaccine theory.

• From its inception in the early 1990s the oral polio vaccine theory had been based on one clear fact—the geographic overlap of the vaccine trials, early AIDS cases, and a high incidence of HIV-1 in the Ruzizi Valley area of DRC, Rwanda, and Burundi. At the meeting Kevin De Cock, an epidemiologist and HIV expert from the Centers for Disease Control and Prevention, working in Nairobi, Kenya, cast doubt on this 'fact'. He described the apparent association as 'ecologic', meaning that although it may be real it was not causal. Formal proof would require that the incidence of HIV/AIDS in polio vaccinees was shown to be significantly greater than in non-vaccinees. But since no records of those vaccinated in the 1950s' trials existed and vaccinees were not followed up, it was impossible to obtain this information. De Cock also questioned the uniqueness of the high incidence of HIV/AIDS in the immediate area of the Ruzizi Valley. This was based on twenty-nine possible early AIDS cases reported in the medical literature and identified by Hooper in *The River*. As De Cock pointed out, DRC is a country the size of Western Europe, which by the mid 1980s had only around 400 hospitals and 1,200 doctors. In this situation only academically minded physicians would have had the time and support to write up such cases, even if they stood out from the background of infectious diseases in the country. So the twenty-nine possible cases reported must represent only a tiny fraction of the total number in the country at the time. He also noted that many of the twenty-nine cases were in towns situated along the Congo River, which in the 1950s acted as a 2,700 km long thoroughfare through DRC. Thus an alternative explanation for the distribution of these cases was that the social mix in these towns at the time was conducive to the rapid spread of HIV-1.

After two days of frank, and at times fraught, discussion, it fell to Robin Weiss, an internationally renowned retrovirologist from University College London, UK, to sum up the proceedings and provide some closing remarks. In carefully chosen words, he concluded that, although at one time the oral polio vaccine theory had been plausible, the weight of scientific evidence now suggested that it was not the means by which HIV-1 entered humans. However, he admitted that such a disastrous event *could* have occurred, and ended by saying: 'Exactly how, when and where the first human(s) became infected with the progenitor of HIV-1 group M, which gave rise to the pandemic strain, is likely, however, to remain a matter of conjecture'.[20]

So, after all the discussion and debate we were still left weighing up probabilities. These had clearly swung in favour of the cut-hunter theory. Virtually all now believed that the oral polio vaccine theory was untenable. But not so Hooper. He and a small band of believers continue to fight their corner, mainly through postings on their websites,[21] still insistent that the theory is plausible and that a scientific conspiracy denies them a fair hearing.

De Cock, referring to the intensity of Hooper's belief, provided a pertinent quote from the late biologist and writer, Sir Peter Medawar: 'the intensity of conviction that a hypothesis is true has no bearing on whether it is true or not'.[22]

*　*　*

Since the year 2000 several new pieces of evidence have emerged that help to tie up the loose ends and in doing so have finally sounded the death knell for the oral polio vaccine theory. Key to this are the studies of Hahn, Sharp, and Peeters identifying ancestral HIV-1 group M in chimpanzees in south-east Cameroon (chapter 4) and Worobey's uncovering of a second virus fossil, DR60, in Kinshasa dating from 1960. This pinpointed the date of virus transfer to near the beginning of the 20th century, certainly no later than the 1930s (chapter 5).

In 2001, stored samples of the actual 40-year-old CHAT vaccine, pool 13, used in the oral polio vaccine campaign in DRC in the late 1950s were located and tested. These proved to contain DNA from Old World monkeys but were entirely negative for SIVs and chimpanzee DNA.[23] Also in 2001, Andrew Rambaut and his colleagues from the University of Oxford, UK, produced evidence to show that the starburst-like evolution of the HIV-1 group M subtypes occurred *after* the ancestral virus's crucial leap from chimpanzee to human. Looking at several hundred viral sequences of the extraordinarily diverse HIV-1 group M viruses from DRC that Peeters originally used to identify Kinshasa as the epicentre of the pandemic,[24] they found that those belonging to the ten or so virus subtypes now recognized were lost in the background of incredible virus diversity. This contrasted with everywhere else in the world where just a few subtypes tend to predominate in any one geographic area. Rambaut concluded that the starburst of subtypes was created in the 1940s or 1950s by individual HIV-1 group M viruses leaving Kinshasa to seed epidemics in other places. Through founder effects, each of these viruses established a new subtype like, for instance, the single HIV-1 group M lineage that travelled from Kinshasa to Haiti around 1966, and on to the

US approximately three years later, to give rise to HIV-1 subgroup B (see chapter 5). Similar events occurred around the world but in Kinshasa no starburst was evident. The uniquely diverse pool of viruses there just continued to evolve so that by the late 1950s, when CHAT was being made and tested, several hundreds of virus strains existed in DRC. For the oral polio vaccine theory to be correct each one of these would have had to be transmitted to humans via the vaccine. As Rambaut states in his letter to *Nature* reporting the findings: 'the HIV-1 sequences from the Congo are evidence that the claim of the OPV [oral polio vaccine] theory that it is "probably the only hypothesis that can readily explain the starburst phenomenon" is incorrect'.[25]

Finally, in 2004 Worobey and co-workers published a letter in *Nature* boldly entitled 'Contaminated polio vaccine theory refuted'. In this they compared SIVs in the urine and faecal samples from wild chimpanzees that he and Hamilton had collected in the Parisi Forest near Kisangani with SIV isolates from *P. t. schweinfurthii* chimpanzees collected by members of Hahn's research group from Gombe National Park in Tanzania. These viruses all clustered together in the evolutionary tree and were quite distinct from SIVs from *P. t. troglodytes* and the HIV group. This confirms that SIVs carried by chimpanzees local to Camp Lindi are not the ancestors of the HIV-1 group of viruses.[26]

* * *

With all this evidence to hand, but still no direct proof for any particular theory, readers must make up their own minds about the way the first HIV-1 group M entered the human population. Personally, like all other scientists I know, I back the cut-hunter theory and will continue to do so unless or until a more plausible hypothesis comes along. However, the alternative name, the 'natural transmission' theory seems more appropriate as it then includes the possibility of the viruses having jumped at any stage of bush meat preparation or even through a bite from a pet chimpanzee. But whatever the name, even this theory leaves several questions unanswered. For instance, why did HIV/AIDS first surface in Leopoldville, DRC, when chimpanzees carrying ancestral HIV-1 group M viruses reside in the Cameroon? Since hunting is an ancient means of obtaining food, why did the HIVs only appear in the late 19th and 20th century and then cross the species barrier on at least twelve separate occasions? How did HIV-1 group M succeed in spreading globally while HIV-1 groups O, N, and P have remained local to Cameroon?

These questions are the subject of the following chapters.

7

The Epic Journey Begins

The revelation that chimpanzees of the subspecies *P.t.troglodytes* carrying ancestral HIV-1 group M reside in the south-east corner of the Cameroon was a landmark in understanding the origins of the pandemic virus. Yet in the years following the momentous discovery of HIV-1 in 1983, another eleven HIVs were isolated, each representing a separate jump from simians to humans. While HIV-1 groups N, O, and P, as well as M viruses, probably all transferred from SIV-carrying chimpanzees (or gorillas) somewhere within their range in the Cameroon, Gabon, the Republic of Congo, or DRC, the eight HIV-2 groups (A to H) did not. They all evolved from SIV_{smm} carried by sooty mangabeys that live over 2,000 kilometres away in West Africa. So although this chapter is mainly concerned with exploring the early history of the pandemic virus HIV-1 group M, any theory relating to its emergence must also explain the extraordinary co-incident appearance of eleven other HIVs, all in the 20th century.

The fact that all HIVs discovered so far are native to west or west central Africa raises questions about the importance of these areas in establishing the viruses in humans. Could there be something unique to this region of Africa in the 20th century that facilitated the jump of SIVs to, and their spread in, humans? Many suggestions have been made, particularly regarding the social changes brought about by colonialism in the late 19th century and the effects of World War I in the early 20th that might have resulted in increased exposure to virus-carrying primates. These include the availability of guns for hunting large game and the granting of logging concessions that opened up previously inaccessible areas of forest. In addition, forced labour took men away from their homes, so necessitating bush meat hunting rather than traditional village-based agriculture.[1] At this stage it is impossible to prove that any of these changes were actually instrumental in the vital interspecies transmissions, but important clues to unravelling these mysterious events are to be found in the natural and social history and geography of west central Africa.

Sub-Saharan Africa is home to a large number of non-human primate species, many of which live, and are regularly hunted for food in west central Africa. Most of these species carry their own strains of retroviruses, and in order to take a closer look at this virus reservoir scientists began by investigating the viruses carried by wild primates living in the Cameroon. One of these, called simian foamy virus, is known to cross the species barrier to infect humans. Named after the frothy appearance it produces in the cells it infects, this virus spreads naturally between juvenile animals via saliva and causes no harm to its natural hosts. The infection is ubiquitous in African and Asian apes and monkeys living in captivity, and several published reports document transfer of simian foamy virus to animal handlers such as zoo and laboratory workers. In one study of over 200 blood samples from North

American animal handlers four tested positive for the virus. All four workers had been bitten or injured in some way by a captive primate or a contaminated instrument.[2] Just like the SIVs, the simian foamy virus' genome sequences differ slightly between their host primate species, and so researchers could distinguish between them. In doing so they were able to ascertain that these infections came from an African green monkey in one case and from baboons in the other three. Thankfully, although simian foamy virus infects humans and establishes a persistent infection, it appears to be non-pathogenic.

Simian foamy virus infection is also common among wild primates and so scientists set about looking for evidence of 'natural' simian foamy virus transfer from primates to humans as a marker of the potential for infection with the less transmissible SIVs. They tested over 1,000 people from nine villages in the Cameroon, all of whom had direct contact with fresh, non-human primate blood, mainly through hunting and butchering the animals. Among these, ten had evidence of simian foamy virus infection.[3] Simian foamy virus sequences amplified from the blood of three of the ten revealed that they each carried a different simian foamy virus—one from a gorilla, one from a mandrill, and one from De Brazza's guenon—all animals indigenous to the study area. This confirms that the present level of contact between humans and primates afforded by hunting and preparing bush meat allows primate viruses to infect humans fairly regularly in west central Africa. Since primates, SIVs, and hunters have co-existed in this area for thousands of years it seems reasonable to suppose that in addition to simian foamy viruses, SIVs have jumped from hunted to hunter here several times in the past.

To assess the size of the SIV reservoir in the wild and its potential threat to humans, Martine Peeters and colleagues tested primate bush meat from over 500 animals caught in the rainforests of Cameroon and on sale at markets in Yaoundé and the surrounding villages. They found SIVs in the majority of primate species they tested, with an infection rate in each ranging from 5 to 40 per cent.[4] This leaves no doubt that a potentially hazardous reservoir exists in the wild, but apart from those SIVs ancestral to the HIV-1 and HIV-2 groups of viruses, there is little evidence that any of these viruses have jumped to humans. We know that several SIVs, including SIV_{cpz} from the eastern chimpanzee, *P.t. schweinfurthii*, are capable of infecting human CD4 T cells in the laboratory but this simple test hardly begins to reproduce the complex processes involved in infecting a whole individual. In one study scientists hunting for proof of natural human SIV infection tested over 6,500 HIV-antibody positive blood samples taken from people living in the Cameroon and Gabon. They found just one possible candidate. The antibodies in this sample reacted more strongly with proteins from a mandrill SIV than with those from either HIV-1 or HIV-2. This suggested that the person, known only as a healthy, 65-year-old male, was infected with the mandrill virus. A similar study found antibodies reactive with SIV proteins in around 17 per cent of seventy-six samples from people who hunted, handled, or butchered non-human primates or kept them as pets. One participant had antibodies strongly reactive with SIV from the eastern black and white colobus monkey. This was tantalizing news, but unfortunately no virus sequences could be amplified from the positive blood samples in either study to confirm the infections.[5, 6]

* * *

Theoretically there are three possible outcomes of an SIV's jump to a cut hunter. The SIV may fail to establish an infection entirely, it may succeed in the short term but be eliminated by the host's immune response, or it may manage to set up a persistent infection. Even if an infection is established the virus may be unable to spread to others; all these alternatives represent 'dead end' infections for which the result is the same—eventual extinction of the virus. On the other hand, if the virus has the potential to infect and spread to others it may create a small focus of infected people. But for a virus to survive long term in humans it must establish a never ending chain of infected hosts, and to reach epidemic proportions each of those infected must on average pass the virus on to more than one other to give an ever expanding population of infected people.

Clearly epidemic expansion requires a large population of susceptible hosts and an efficient method of virus spread between them. This may be easy for viruses like flu and measles that spread rapidly and widely via air currents, but for the HIVs it is not. Back in the early 1900s the HIVs' only transmission route was directly from one host to another, either via blood or sexual contact, and the viruses could only go where their hosts took them. The most likely scenario is that the cut hunter lived in a traditional African village in rural Cameroon where opportunities for spread between hosts must have been very limited. In this setting most SIVs that jumped to humans would have been unable to maintain a chain of infection and died out unrecognized. This would probably have included all the HIVs if they had jumped to humans over 150 years ago. Indeed, although they have been recognized in humans, the non-epidemic HIV-1 groups N and P fall into this category even today. In order to thrive, these viruses must gain access to a large population, and one event that might have provided an HIV-like virus with the opportunity to spread beyond its homeland prior to the 20th century is the slave trade.

*   *   *

From the 15th century onwards Europeans regularly traded along the west coast of Africa, acquiring highly desirable luxury goods such as gold and ivory as well as buying slaves when the opportunity arose for onward sale. But slave trading was just a minor concern until everything changed in 1492 when Columbus's transatlantic voyage opened up the Americas to European exploitation. For the next 300 years the inexhaustible demand for slave labour from the sugar plantations of the Caribbean and South America made this a highly lucrative business. Transatlantic traffic of human cargo rose exponentially. By 1867, when the trade was nearing its end, around 11 million people had been exported from Africa to the Americas, and countless millions had lost their lives before the voyage even began.

This forced, mass human migration gave microbes the opportunity to cross the Atlantic for the first time. Parasites that cause tropical diseases like malaria, river blindness, schistosomiasis, and elephantiasis colonized the Americas, as did certain viruses. Yellow fever virus, for instance, survived the transatlantic voyage by serially infecting those on board slave ships, spread between them by mosquitoes that bred in casks of drinking water carried on board. Long-distance travel was much easier for blood-borne viruses like hepatitis B, since it establishes a persistent infection with a long silent period. Thus it could reach the New World inside slaves. Even more relevant to HIV is the retrovirus, human T cell leukaemia virus (HTLV)-I, discovered just before HIV-1 in the early 1980s. Like the HIVs, this virus sets up a persistent infection of CD4 T cells and spreads by blood and sexual contact. HTLV-I infection is either entirely asymptomatic or induces leukaemia several decades after the initial infection. Scientists postulate that HTLV-I also has its origins in Africa where it probably jumped from simians to humans on several occasions around 20,000 years ago. Slaves carried this virus to the Caribbean where it established a focus of infection that still exists today.

Available records suggest that around 800,000 slaves were shipped from the area of west central Africa that is now the Cameroon, Gabon, and DRC, and covers the range of ancestral HIV-1-carrying chimpanzees.[7] In reality this figure may have been a great deal higher, and so *if* a predecessor to the HIVs had been around at the time it *could* have found its way across the Atlantic where it *may* have thrived in this massive social upheaval. But this is all hypothetical as there is no evidence that such a virus reached the Americas before HIV-1 group M, subtype B, was introduced to the people of Haiti in the mid 1960s. Thus we have established as best we can that despite the coincidence of hunting primates and SIVs in west central Africa for millennia, SIV/HIV infection was either extremely rare or non-existent in the local population prior to the early 20th century. Consequently, we are seeking a unique event or set of circumstances that occurred in the late 19th and/or early 20th century, which facilitated SIVs' jumps to humans, enabled HIV-1 group M's initial local expansion, and prompted its exodus from the Cameroon—the first steps in its global journey.

Viruses that succeed in transferring to, and surviving in, a new host generally undergo a period of rapid adaptation. During this time their 'fitness' improves, meaning that they hone their survival skills so that they can infect, evade host immunity, and spread between the new hosts more efficiently. Like any other organism adapting to an alien environment, this is accomplished by the Darwinian process of mutation and natural selection. Only the best adapted, or fittest, viruses are transmitted along the chain of infection. But as the HIVs' genomes mutate so much faster than mammalian DNA—so their adaptation can also be fast. However, since no one knows how many mutations were required for $SIV_{cpz-Ptt}$ to become fully fledged HIV-1, we cannot estimate exactly how long this process would have taken.

Scientists trying to model SIV's adaptation to a new host infected captive pig-tailed macaques (*Macaca nemestrina*) with a hybrid SIV_{mac} (called SHIV) in which the SIV *env* gene had been replaced by *env* from HIV-1.[8] This means that all the properties of SHIV's Env protein, including binding to and infecting host cells and mutating rapidly to evade the host's immune response, were derived from HIV-1 *env* in the hybrid virus. The scientists had already ascertained that SHIV caused no symptoms in infected macaques, and as expected the first pair of infected animals remained healthy. But still the scientists rescued virus-infected cells from these macaques and injected them into a second pair of animals. They then took virus-infected cells from the second pair to infect a third pair of animals and so on, eventually passing the virus through five pairs of animals. As the experiment progressed the virus became increasingly adapted to its new host. In the first two groups it grew poorly in the hosts' CD4 T cells and consequently no disease ensued, but the outcome for the animals in groups three, four, and five was dramatically different. The virus grew well in these animals and they rapidly developed high virus loads and low CD4 T cell counts. Within a year three of the six animals had clear signs of AIDS, the result of selecting a fast growing virus strain that wiped out their CD4 T cells. Although this experimental design is far removed from the natural setting in which the HIVs evolved, it does give some indication of how rapidly SIVs can adapt to a new host. But the question is, could $SIV_{cpz-Ptt}$ have evolved naturally into the virulent HIV-1 group M we know today in the rural population of southeast Cameroon?

For one group of scientists headed by Preston Marx from Tulane Primate Research Center, Louisiana, the answer to this question is definitely no. They believe that under natural circumstances a poorly replicating SIV would be eliminated by the human immune response before it had time to adapt. To investigate the dynamics of HIV's adaptation they devised a computer model that predicted the time taken for SIV_{cpz} to become HIV-1 using a range of different values for the (unknown) number of mutations it might require. The computer came up with a prediction of 65 days if 100 mutations are required for a poorly-replicating SIV to mutate into HIV-1 in its new human host and 80 days if 200 mutations are needed. As the human immune response takes only around ten days to reach its peak, this result led the scientists to state that they had found that:

> the emergence of even one epidemic HIV strain following a single exposure to SIV, was very unlikely. And the probability of four or more such transitions (i.e [the epidemic viruses] HIV-1 groups M, O and HIV-2 groups A and B) occurring in a brief period is vanishingly small.[9]

They suggested that in order to evolve into an epidemic HIV-1 or HIV-2 virus, the ancestral SIV would have needed a helping hand. They postulated that this came from human intervention in the form of mass treatment and vaccination campaigns that were undertaken in Africa in the early 20th century. Simply stated their theory is that serial human passage of SIV by contamination of unsterile injection equipment enabled the emergence of epidemic HIVs in Africa. I should stress at this point that this theory is very different from the now out-dated oral polio vaccine theory discussed in the previous chapter that invokes SIV_{cpz} contaminated polio vaccine delivery as the route of transmission of SIV_{cpz} from chimpanzees to humans. In contrast, Marx and colleagues accept the cut hunter theory for the initial virus transfer. But they argue that this first infection could not have persisted in the cut hunter for long enough for the virus to spread onwards via the sexual route before it had fully adapted to its new host. So the only way that these viruses could have kept one step ahead of the immune response while the adaptation process was ongoing was by being picked up directly from the bloodstream and moved on during the early acute stage of the disease when the blood viral load is high and before immune cells were aware of their presence. Given the rapidity with which HIV-1 passed between needle-sharing intravenous drug users in the US and Europe in the early 1980s, and is still doing so today in certain parts of the world, there is no doubt that unsterile needles are a very effective means of virus transmission. But do the historical facts support the theory?

* * *

The hypodermic syringe was invented in 1848; a handmade glass and metal instrument so costly that for several decades its use was very restricted even in the Western world. Far from being the cheap, disposable, plastic device we know today, this valuable piece of medical equipment was designed to be sterilized in boiling water and reused many times. Of course, as the demand for syringes rose, manufacture was stepped up and cheaper options became available (Figure 17). During the 1920s, global production rose from 100,000 to over 2 million, but it was the advent of penicillin (initially only available in injectable form) in the late 1940s that prompted the massive demand that forced change. By 1950, 7.5 million syringes were produced annually and when shortly thereafter the first disposable syringes reached the market the price dropped to US 1.5 cents per unit. Global production hit a billion in 1960.[10]

In parallel with the explosion in syringe use in the Western world, several mass treatment and vaccination campaigns got under way in Africa in the early decades of the 20th century. From

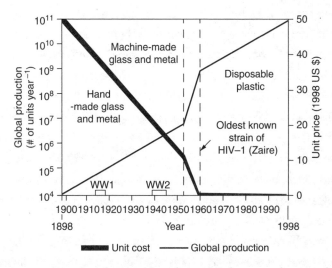

FIGURE 17 Diagram showing the relationship between the growth of global production of injecting equipment and the unit cost between 1898 and 1998.

Source: From Marx PA et al, *Phil Trans R Soc B*, 356: 911–920 (2001), by permission of the Royal Society.

that time onwards Belgians, French, British, German, Portuguese, and Spanish authorities in west central Africa treated hundreds of thousands of sufferers of common diseases like malaria, syphilis, yaws, tuberculosis, and leprosy using injectable drugs. As in the West, the biggest boost to syringe use in Africa came with the new antibiotics from the 1950s onwards. One example was the United Nations campaign for the eradication of yaws, a chronic bacterial skin infection associated with poverty and poor hygiene, which was extremely common in African children from rural areas. The campaign began in the early 1950s and treated around 35 million children. We will never know how many of these millions of injections were given with unsterile equipment but since a sleeping sickness campaign in 1917–1919 in the Central African Republic is purported to have screened around 90,000 people and treated over 5,000 cases using only six syringes, it is highly likely that on occasions blood-borne viruses were transmitted along with the life-saving drugs.

It is difficult to relate this information directly to the emergence of HIVs but there are certainly several precedents for viruses being spread by the treatment campaigns of the early 20th century. The largest and best documented of these is transmission of the persistent, blood-borne hepatitis C virus (HCV) during the massive campaign to eradicate schistosomiasis in Egypt. This began in 1920 and ran continuously until 1980. Schistosomiasis is a potentially fatal disease caused by a parasitic blood fluke that is spread between victims by water snails living in slow-flowing fresh water courses. The irrigation channels used by farmers along the River Nile are close to ideal for these snails and thus at the time Egypt had the highest rates of schistosomiasis in the world. The first available treatment for the disease was potassium antimony tartrate or 'tartar emetic', administered to sufferers in

Egypt for most of the sixty years by a course of twelve to sixteen intravenous injections. At its height between 1966 and 1969 the intensive treatment campaign delivered three million injections to around 250,000 sufferers annually.[11]

It was only in the 1990s that Egypt's huge burden of liver disease caused by HCV was uncovered. Around one in five Egyptians carry the virus but it is the clear co-incidence of the highest levels of HCV infection with those of past schistosomiasis that identified the treatment campaign as the culprit. HCV infection rates are 28 per cent among the farming communities of the Nile Delta while in the cities of Cairo and Alexandria where schistosomiasis had always been rare, rates are just 6–8 per cent. Also, HCV infection rates rise with age, peaking at 55 per cent in the oldest age group in the Delta area; the group that would have been young, working adults at the height of the campaign.

A WHO report from 1964 states that: 'the skilful doctor began injecting at 9.20 a.m. and completed 504 injections of men, women and children by 10.10 a.m. Allowing for a 10-min rest, the time taken for each injection was thus just under 5s...The used syringe is placed in an 'out' tray, from which it is taken by a nurse, washed thoroughly and boiled for a minute or two...There are usually 20 to 30 syringes in rotation.'[12] It does not take much imagination to realize that any slight mishap would disrupt this tight schedule, so allowing unsterile syringes to slip through. In any case, we now know that one or two minutes in boiling water is not adequate to ensure that HIV is inactivated.

Sadly, collecting similar data on HIV-1 group M infection rates in areas of Africa where mass treatment and prevention campaigns took place in the early 20th century is not possible because anyone infected during one of these campaigns would have long since died of AIDS. However, in two parallel studies in west central Africa scientists used the blood-borne viruses HCV and HTLV-I as proxy for HIV-1 since infection with these viruses is compatible with long-term survival of the host. Both studies were conducted in rural areas close to the range of SIV$_{cpz-Ptt}$ carrying chimpanzees. The first was in southern Cameroon where HCV infection rates are second only to those in Egypt. Fifty-six per cent of the study participants were HCV positive and scientists found that the risk of infection was highest in older people and those who had received intravenous treatment for malaria. Furthermore, molecular clock analysis of HCV isolates suggested a period of exponential growth coincident with the treatment programme in the first half of the 20th century.[13] The second study looked at HTLV-I infection in inhabitants of a group of villages in the Central African Republic close to the border with south-east Cameroon where sleeping sickness was highly prevalent between 1936 and 1950. This identified a link between HTLV-I infection and treatment or prevention of sleeping sickness.[14] Interestingly, using existing colonial records from the treatment campaign, the scientists predicted that about 60 per cent of the study participants who were 65 or older would have been treated for sleeping sickness in the 1950s. In fact only 11 per cent reported suffering from the disease and receiving the treatment. The scientists suggested that this large discrepancy was due to many of those treated for sleeping sickness acquiring HIV-1 group M along with the drugs and dying prematurely from AIDS. Be that as it may, these two studies certainly support the suggestion that blood-borne viruses were unwittingly spread to masses of people by unsterile needles in the very area, and at around the same time as the HIV-1 viruses are thought to have emerged. HIV-1 may very well have been among them, but the scientists go further. They postulate that initially SIV_{cpz} in a lone carrier was picked up and serially passed from one person to another. This helped it to adapt to its new host while generating a pool of HIV-1 group M infected people large enough to sustain dissemination via the sexual route. However, although these studies provide circumstantial evidence for the early spread of HIV-1 group M via contaminated medical equipment, they stop short of proving that this was an essential step in the virus's adaptation to its new human host. Unfortunately, now, many decades later, it is not possible to prove or disprove this theory for any of the epidemic HIVs, and so we will move on to the next stage of HIV-1 group M's journey—its exit from the Cameroon.

*   *   *

The crucial discoveries of the unprecedented level of virus diversity and of the two earliest virus isolates, ZR59 and DR60, in Kinshasa, DRC, pointed the finger at this city as the epicentre of the pandemic. So in order to make any sense of HIV-1 group M's early history we must first bridge the gap between its birthplace in south-east Cameroon and its global launch pad in Kinshasa.

As discussed in chapter 5, the best estimate for the timing of the most recent common ancestor for HIV-1 group M viruses calculated from the genetic distance between the fossil viruses, ZR59 and DRC60, is somewhere between 1884 and 1924.[15] So HIV-1 must have first infected the person who introduced it to Kinshasa at some time between these two dates. It is highly improbable that this was the original cut hunter, but someone, or a series of people, carried the virus from south-east Cameroon to Kinshasa. In discussing their work on the emergence of HIV-1 group M, Sharp, Hahn, and Worobey have all stressed the coincidence of the virus's emergence and the rise of large colonial cities in west central Africa. They suggest that these urban conurbations were in some way essential for the virus's survival and expansion, and so investigating the colonial history of the region may turn up possible triggers for HIV-1 group M's pandemic spread.

In 1884 Cameroon came under the control of the German government with Chancellor Bismarck at the helm. The Germans immediately set about developing road and rail networks and a port on the Atlantic coast at Douala with a view to exploiting the country's potential wealth—ivory, rubber, timber, coffee and cocoa—to the full. Then, at the onset of World War I, the British marched into Cameroon from Nigeria while the French invaded from French Equatorial Africa, and the Germans retreated. At the end of the war the country was divided between the French and British with the French acquiring the lion's share, French Cameroon, including the area of interest in south-eastern Cameroon where HIV-1 group M was born.

French colonials further developed the port of Douala and, although Yaoundé became the capital city in 1916 because of its more central location in the country, Douala remained the largest city and the commercial centre. Yet compared to Kinshasa (then called Leopoldville), even by the mid 1900s Douala was still a relatively small city that attracted few migrants. In most of the country traditional African village culture prevailed, and this was particularly true of the remote, densely forested, south-eastern corner of the Cameroon. Here the main trading route and thoroughfare was the Sangha River, a tributary of the great Congo River.

The Congo River basin occupies over four million square kilometres of central and west Africa, with the river running for 4,700 km from its source in the East African Rift mountains to its estuary on the Gulf of Guinea. Although a series of falls or rapids, known as the Stanley Falls, render the river unnavigable between the Atlantic coast and the interior, beyond the falls is the Malebo Pool with Kinshasa on the south side and Brazzaville, capital of the Republic of Congo, on the north. From here a constant flow of river traffic heads both between the two capital cities and up and down the main river and its tributaries, penetrating the otherwise impenetrable forest and providing the region's main transportation system.

We shall never know exactly how HIV-1 group M travelled from south-east Cameroon to Leopoldville, but since at the time there were no roads in the area and the main towns of Yaoundé and Douala were several hundred kilometres away, it seems most likely that the virus travelled along the Sangha River, perhaps via its tributaries. In a journey of some 700 kilometres it would have passed along the border between the Cameroon and the Republic of Congo and then across the Republic to meet the Congo River at its border with the DRC as the river flowed down to Leopoldville (Figure 18a). Whether the virus made it in a single leap inside someone heading straight for Leopoldville or in several short hops, perhaps carried from one fishing community to another by visiting river traders, somehow it reached Leopoldville in the early 20th century. Thereafter it was the unique series of social upheavals in Leopoldville that determined the fate of the virus and eventually affected the whole world.

The history of the DRC is very different from that of neighbouring Cameroon and the Republic of Congo and a short summary seems appropriate here. The Portuguese were the first

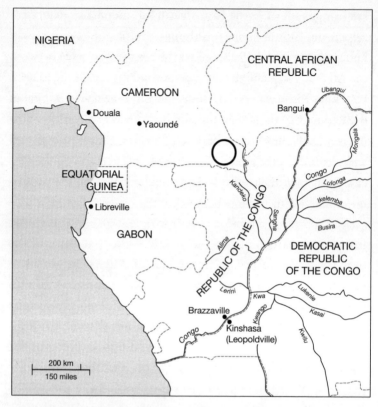

FIGURE 18a Map of west-central Africa showing the Congo River and its tributaries. Also shown are the major cities with explosive population growth in the 20th century. The circle marks the location of chimpanzees carrying SIV$_{cpz}$ most closely related to HIV-1.
Source: Figure 1a in Sharp and Hahn Nature 455: 605–606. 2008.

outsiders known to have visited the area as their exploration of the west coast of Africa took them into the estuary of the Congo River in the 15th century. There they met the Kongo people, from whom the name of the country derives, living on its banks. For a few decades the Portuguese and the Kongo people traded amicably, some of the latter even visiting Portugal and adopting the Christian faith. But all this changed in the 16th century when European slave traders plundered the area.

*   *   *

Following the slave traders came European explorers intent on opening up the interior of the region that is now DRC and mapping its geography. Early visitors sailing up the Congo River from the sea were deterred by the rapids, while further inland it was tropical diseases that took their toll. Consequently, this was one of the last regions in Africa to be penetrated by Europeans. The man who eventually succeeded was the British-born, American journalist cum explorer, Henry Morton Stanley. His first visit to Africa, financed by the *New York Herald*, was in search of the famous British missionary and explorer, David Livingstone, who had gone missing somewhere in central Africa in the late 1860s. Stanley set off from Zanzibar Island off the coast of East Africa in 1871 and found Livingstone living contentedly in a village near the eastern shores of Lake Tanganyika (prompting the famous 'Doctor Livingstone I presume') and not inclined to go home. Both men were driven by the explorer's dream of finding the source of the Nile, and together they ascertained that Lake Tanganyika was *not* the source before Stanley headed home to write a book on his travels that was to make his name as an explorer. Stanley set out for Africa in 1874, again backed by the newspaper, this time to track the course of the Lualaba River. He thought that perhaps it would lead him to the Nile but in fact it is a tributary of the Congo River. Despite enormous hardship he and his party of 356 men followed the sweep of the great river northwards and then to the south-west through dense jungle for 999 days before arriving at Boma trading station at the mouth of the river in 1877. Over two-thirds of the men were lost en route either deserting the party or dying from disease or starvation, while he and the remaining men arrived just days away from death themselves.

Stanley's epic journey was a turning point in the history of the DRC. He was well aware of the great potential of the land he had travelled through and his aim was to profit from it. While Britain was not interested in the prospect of colonization, King Leopold II of Belgium certainly was. Within two years Stanley was back in the DRC laying claim to the huge area, called the Congo Free State, as King Leopold's own personal colony.

In one of the worst cases of exploitation and brutality by a colonial power, between 1885 and 1908 Leopold proceeded to milk this huge central African colony of its riches, including rubber, ivory, and wood, for his own personal gain. He employed forced labour to build roads and railways as well as for mining, harvesting, and carrying goods. During the twenty-three years of Leopold's ownership the country's population dropped dramatically as people were killed, died of disease, or fled the inhumane regime. It is interesting to reflect that this was the time when the Polish-born British author, Joseph Conrad, was in the Congo Free State, sent there to replace a steamship captain who had been killed by tribesmen. Appalled by the brutality he witnessed, Conrad's novel *The Heart of Darkness* is based on his experiences. By the time the novel was published in 1902 news of the atrocities carried out in the name of King Leopold had already alarmed other European nations. They commissioned a report, the damning nature of which ensured that the Congo Free State was dissolved. In 1908 its ownership was transferred to the Belgian government and the country became the Belgian Congo. Following this transfer of power the lot of the Congolese people improved, but the majority of the country's riches continued to flow to Belgium and a system based on racism and exploitation remained. Even by 1960 when the country became independent it is reputed that only 17 of the 14 million Congolese in the country had received a university education and there were no doctors among them.

In 1881 Stanley established a trading post on the site of a former fishing village on the Pool and named it Leopoldville after the Belgian king. Because of its strategic position above the rapids, this quickly became a bustling commercial centre. All incoming and outgoing goods passed through on their way to and from the coast, initially being carried on the heads of hundreds of porters for the 250 kilometres around the rapids to the port of Matadi below. Then, when the Matadi-Leopoldville railway link opened in 1898, Leopoldville became the country's commercial hub and in 1920 it superseded Boma as the capital of the Belgian Congo.

Sometime during the early 1900s HIV-1 group M slipped into Leopoldville unnoticed. It may have been just chance that it arrived here rather than in Brazzaville, capital of the French Congo. The city's position on the opposite side of the Pool was perhaps a more likely destination for someone coming from the Cameroon. Indeed, it is possible that the virus *did* first arrive in Brazzaville as a recent study of modern virus isolates from Brazzaville shows that they are just as diverse as those in Kinshasa.[16] Unfortunately, no fossil HIV-1 viruses have been found in Brazzaville to help uncover its early history. In any case, the constant traffic between the twin cities would have ensured that any virus was transported back and forth between them several times during its early life. And there is little doubt that at the time Leopoldville provided the best chance of survival for the virus and for its later epidemic expansion. While Brazzaville was the capital of a resource-poor country and remained mainly an administrative centre, Leopoldville was the

(b)

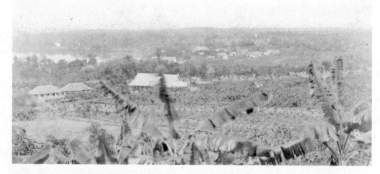

(c)

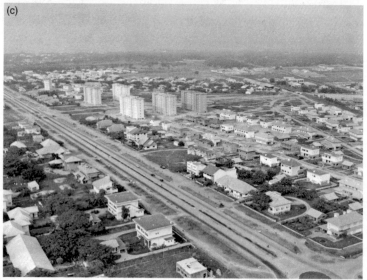

FIGURE 18b, 18c Leopoldville in 1905(b) and 1955(c).
©INTERFOTO/Alamy.

capital of a wealthy country rich in natural resources. With diamonds, copper, cobalt, tin, zinc, manganese, and even uranium all being mined, and rubber and coffee grown on a huge scale, it rapidly became a boom town (Figure 18b and c).

At the turn of the 20th century Leopoldville had a population of around 10 thousand, twice that of Brazzaville, and rising rapidly. As huge influxes of migrant workers arrived, coerced into private industrial work and public building projects, the population rose from 16,000 in 1920 to 47,000 in 1929. Then, following a fall coincident with the world recession of the 1930s, it reached 200,000 by 1950 and double that by the 1960s. Perhaps the first HIV-1 group M virus arrived in the city inside one of the migrant workers, and having done so found a unique situation that allowed it to thrive.

Probably one of the most important factors in HIV-1 group M's survival was the Belgian policy of conscripting men into a massive labour force while discouraging their wives and families from leaving their villages. This caused a huge gender imbalance in the main towns and cities, and nowhere was it more pronounced than in Leopoldville. Here male predominance reached a peak in the late 1920s when they outnumbered females by over 4:1. Unsurprisingly this encouraged commercial sex and caused unprecedentedly high levels of sexually transmitted diseases. And the very social factors that allowed these established infections to thrive also encouraged the spread of a new, hidden STD—HIV-1 group M. But there was more. Pre-existing sexually transmitted disease, particularly those that cause genital ulcers, dramatically increases the risk of HIV transmission between sexual partners. Early African studies showed that genital ulcer disease in female commercial sex workers increased the risk of HIV-1 male to female transmission 10–50 times per sexual act and 50–300 times for female to male transmission.[17]

In contrast, male circumcision was found to reduce the risk of HIV-1 transmission quite dramatically. In one study in men who acquired genital ulcer disease from commercial sex workers, the concomitant HIV-1 transmission rates were 43 per cent per sexual act in the non-circumcised group compared to 4 per cent in the circumcised participants.[18] These massive infection rates, which are only exceeded by transfusion-related HIV-1 transmission, combined with the widespread genital ulcer disease in Africa, led experts to conclude that over half of the new infections in Africa occur via genital ulcer disease-assisted virus transmission.

With this in mind, a group of scientists from the University of Leuven, Belgium, used old official colonial health reports and articles in medical journals to assess the incidence of genital ulcer disease in large colonial cities of west central Africa within the range of *P.t.troglodytes* chimpanzees, including Leopoldville, Brazzaville, and Douala.[19] Between 1890 and 1920 the most common infections causing genital ulcers were syphilis and chancroid. These are both caused by bacteria which produce ulcers that persist and remain infectious for around five months in the former and ten weeks in the latter. Both diseases were probably introduced to west central Africa by Europeans when they arrived in the late 1800s, and the incidence rose dramatically in the social disruption that followed. The effect was most marked in Leopoldville with its rapidly growing population, large migrant worker force and marked male gender bias. A survey in 1928 estimated that nearly half of the 6,000 women in the city were 'mainly living on prostitution'. In colonial terms this included any woman with multiple sexual partners, be they a full-time commercial sex worker or so-called '*femme libres*'—unmarried, working women with a few, regular sexual partners. Large surveys in the early 1930s in Leopoldville revealed that 5 per cent of these women had active genital ulcer disease and the overall incidence of syphilis was 10 per cent. After this revelation, partially successful treatment campaigns and screening of sex workers led to a decline in sexually transmitted diseases in the mid 1930s that continued until independence in 1960.[20] This study also uncovered a lower rate of male circumcision in the early 20th century compared to modern times. Although this was difficult to quantify accurately as it differed between ethnic groups and information about circumcision practices was often incomplete, best estimates suggest that in 1910 around 70–80 per cent of men in Leopoldville were circumcised and this rose steadily, reaching present-day levels of over 95 per cent by 1960. Clearly this lower level of circumcision combined with the high level of genital ulcer disease must have helped HIV-1 group M to become established in Leopoldville's high-risk population. Indeed, using a computer-simulated model of HIV-1 group M emergence in Leopoldville, the same scientists concluded that the virus could not have survived in a pre-colonial village setting due to the absence of commercial sex workers and sexually transmitted diseases. Its best chance of generating a continuous chain of infection in Leopoldville was between 1919 and 1929, the exact period predicted for the arrival of the pandemic virus in the city. But this window of opportunity soon closed as healthcare for at-risk groups improved and levels of sexually transmitted diseases in the city fell, so that if the virus had arrived in 1950 its chances of survival would have been small. Whether the virus really did reach the city and survive under its own steam, meaning by chance, or whether, as other scientists propose, it required an essential boost from contaminated injecting equipment for its initial adaptation, we shall probably never know. In any case the outcome is the same—one way or another the virus maintained a chain of infection that took it to Leopoldville where social changes prompted its epidemic expansion.

* * *

Following independence from Belgian rule and the birth of the DRC in 1960, the much revered ex post office clerk and political activist, Patrice Lumumba, became prime minister of the new state. Hopes were high but unfortunately disaster rapidly followed. With virtually no preparations for the handover of power, the new government had no chance of fulfilling the expectations of the newly liberated population. Within a few months the army mutinied and riots broke out. At this point most of the remaining Belgians fled the violence and the government collapsed. Lumumba was overthrown by the army and its Colonel in Chief, Joseph Mobutu, soon to become the corrupt dictator of the next thirty years, took charge. In a matter of weeks Lumumba was imprisoned, escaped, and was recaptured, and in January 1961 he was executed; just six months after Independence Day. Thereafter civil war ensued and refugees headed for Kinshasa in their thousands. Unemployment in the capital city reached 25 per cent, poverty was rife, and brothels flourished. It is likely that in these chaotic times HIV-1 group M, which had lain low in the city for so long, began its epidemic growth. Having worked its way through local sexual networks the virus then mainly followed trade routes as it moved through central Africa as a prelude to its global journey.

With virtually no Congolese teachers to educate the country's children, or doctors and nurses to treat the sick, the United Nations and the WHO took a hand in providing this essential workforce. Many professionals were recruited from Haiti so that by the mid 1960s several thousand Haitian teachers, doctors, nurses, and technicians were working in the DRC. It is most likely that one of these people carried HIV-1 group M back with them to Haiti, either while on a short visit home or when returning permanently after completing their term of service. Again we shall never know the details, but we do know that just one virus strain inside a single individual seeded the epidemic in Haiti around 1966, and then around 1969 another single strain moved on to the US.

*   *   *

We have now followed HIV-1 group M in a full circle from the first recognition of AIDS in the US in 1981 and the discovery of the virus in 1983 back to its roots in west central Africa at the beginning of the 20th century and its jump from there to the US around 1969. And although some ends are left untied, most of the fine details of this incredible tale of medical detection are complete. But what of the viruses themselves? In the next chapter we look at what the HIVs and SIVs can tell us about why some are pathogenic while others are not, and why some have caused epidemics and pandemics while others have hardly moved from their site of origin.

8

Adapting to Humans

While epidemiologists and evolutionary biologists were busy unravelling the intricacies of the HIVs' birth and first tentative steps, cellular and molecular biologists set about investigating the viruses themselves. They are addressing broader questions about how retroviruses adapt to a new host species and this is still very much work in progress. Hopefully it will provide answers to some unresolved questions. In particular, why just two SIVs have succeeded in infecting humans when we know that bush meat hunters come into contact with many more, and why the SIVs and HIVs differ in their ability to cause disease. More importantly perhaps, scientists are trying to figure out why the four HIV-1 groups that have jumped to humans behave so differently in their new host. How, for instance, has HIV-1 group M managed to infected 60–80 million people in its unstoppable global journey while HIV-1 groups O, N and P have remained local to the Cameroon and Gabon? Currently group O viruses infect around 25,000 people and less than 20 are infected with group N and P viruses. So in this chapter we switch focus from the pandemic to the viruses themselves. We take a close look at their interactions with the cells they infect, and at some exciting recent discoveries that might explain some of these discrepancies.

HIVs evolve rapidly and clearly this is an essential attribute in avoiding eradication by the immune response in each new host they infect. But while the mutations they acquire help to counteract immune mechanisms in one host, they are not necessarily beneficial for spreading to and colonizing the next. These viruses meet a barrier each time they try to move on, such that even when they successfully colonize a new host it is often just one virus particle that establishes the infection. This results in a severe bottleneck at each transmission, causing the founder effect which, as we have seen in chapter 5, spawned an array of HIV-1 group M subtypes that spread to specific geographical locations around the globe. The genome sequences of these subtype viruses now differ from each other by 10–35 per cent, but whether any of the mutations they have accumulated are associated with virus adaptation to humans is not yet clear. If so, we might expect that subtypes would differ in biological properties such as virulence (the rate of host deaths as a result of infection), the length of the lag period before AIDS ensues, or their ability to spread between hosts. Yet information in this area is sparse and there is no firm evidence to suggest that HIV-1 group M's virulence has changed at all over the past thirty years. This is mainly because no cohort studies large enough to provide meaningful answers were set up in the 1980s, and such studies would not be possible today since the drug combination known as highly active anti retroviral therapy (HAART) successfully interrupts the natural progression of the disease.

Some believe that HIV-1 group M subtype C viruses are more transmissible than other subtype viruses. Certainly from a worldwide perspective they have spread more rapidly and in some places have even ousted the resident subtype. Subtype C now accounts for over 50 per cent of HIV-1 infections worldwide, but this could be down to chance—because founder subtype C viruses just happened to be introduced into the huge populations of South Africa and Asia.

Obviously it is important to know how HIV-1 group M is going to behave in the future and it is often said that over tens or perhaps hundreds of years the virus will become less virulent as it adapts to us and we adapt to the virus. This supposition is mainly based on a single observation—the myxomatosis virus 'experiment' undertaken in the 1950s. Myxomatosis virus naturally infects rabbits in Brazil causing a mild illness, but when it was introduced into the wild rabbit populations of Britain and Australia in an attempt to control their numbers, it wiped out 99.8 per cent of those infected. Seven years later only around a quarter of infections proved lethal and eventually most infected animals survived and the rabbit problem was as bad as ever. But this rapid adaptation, presumably of both the rabbits and the virus, does not occur in every situation. A virus is under selection pressure to maximize its spread by replicating at high levels but also to limit the severity of the disease it causes so as not to wipe out its host before it can be passed on. Thus multiple factors are involved in determining virus fitness and not all of them relate to virulence. For instance, in the case of HIV-1, over time a less virulent virus strain may be selected if keeping its host alive for longer provided more opportunities for the virus to spread to others during the long lag period. On the other hand, if a more virulent form of the virus produced a higher viral load during primary infection and consequently spread more effectively despite its host's shorter life span then this variant would be selected. But the evidence is conflicting and so the jury is still out on this one. Based on laboratory experiments suggesting that subtype C viruses replicate less efficiently than other subtype viruses, some argue that they are less virulent, although they seem to be transmitted as efficiently as other subtype viruses. Others have shown that subtype C viruses produce a higher virus load than other subtypes, so pointing to an overall increased virulence. Clearly these contradictory findings require further investigation.[1]

* * *

In 2007 Paul Sharp and colleagues took a molecular approach for seeking mutations that might represent adaptive changes in the HIV-1 group of viruses. They compared genome sequences from viruses ancestral to HIV-1 groups M, N, and O viruses with twelve genome sequences from $SIV_{cpz-Ptt}$. They were searching for specific mutations that produced differences between the chimpanzee and human virus' genomes but were conserved in all viruses from the same species. In the end they came up with just one mutation—at site Gag-30 in the *gag* gene. In SIV_{cpz} Gag-30 codes for the amino acid methionine (Met) but this is swapped for arginine (Arg) in the genomes of the ancestors of all three HIV-1 groups.[2] Met to Arg may sound like a small change but in fact it is quite radical. Met, a neutral, sulphur-containing amino acid, is replace by Arg, a basic one, in what scientists call a 'non-conservative amino acid replacement' to indicate that by changing the overall charge of the protein this could radically alter its shape and function. To give a well-known but non-virological example, the disease sickle cell anaemia is caused by just such a point mutation in the β-globin portion of the vital oxygen-carrying protein, haemoglobin A. When a neutral valine replaces glutamic acid at position six in the amino acid chain, the resulting haemoglobin S variant causes red blood cells to bend into a sickle shape, giving them a short life span and resulting in sickle cell anaemia.

The fact that all three HIV-1 groups of viruses have independently switched from Met to Arg at Gag-30 means that this is highly unlikely to have been a chance event and strongly implies a host-specific adaptation. This supposition was reinforced by study of genome sequences from HIV-1 isolates from two chimpanzees that had been experimentally infected with HIV-1 back in the 1990s during the search for a suitable primate model for AIDS. Both virus isolates turned out to resemble SIV_{cpz} rather than the parent HIV-1 used to infect the chimpanzees, in having switched from Arg to Met at Gag-30. To find out if this mutation had any effect on the biological properties of these two virus isolates, Sharp's group infected human and chimpanzee CD4 T cells with them in the laboratory. Remarkably, the Met-containing viruses grew much better in chimpanzee than human cells, but after the scientists mutated Gag-30 back to the original HIV-1 sequence the resulting viruses grew better in human cells. This indicates a strong selective pressure for Met at Gag-30 when the virus infects chimpanzees. Frustratingly though, we do not know exactly how the Arg to Met mutation affects viral fitness at the functional level. The part of the *gag* gene that contains Gag-30 codes for the virus matrix protein that forms a covering for the virus inside its capsid. It plays an important role in the correct assembly of new viruses in an infected cell, and in doing so it interacts with several host cell proteins. So although the details are yet to be unravelled, it is easy to imagine how disrupting one of these interactions after a jump to a new host might critically affect viral fitness.

Interestingly, alone among the HIV-1 group M subtypes, C viruses have Met at Gag-30. Since this subtype evolved from a group M virus that had already swapped Met for Arg at Gag-30, subtype C founder virus must have undergone a reversion from Arg to Met. Why this should have happened, and how it impacts on the virulence of the subtype we do not know, but it is interesting that, as discussed above, subtype C, while a highly successful spreader, may differ in virulence from other subtype viruses.

* * *

As outlined in chapter 1, much to everyone's amazement, when the full human genome sequence project was completed in 2003 it revealed remnants of ancient retrovirus genomes that accounted for 8 per cent of the total DNA—more than all the protein-coding gene sequences put together. This provides good evidence that our ancestors suffered from retrovirus infections, and that these have been instrumental in driving the evolution of retaliatory measures. The battle between retroviruses and their primate hosts has clearly been ongoing for millions of years as both invader and invaded have evolved ever more sophisticated manoeuvres to counteract each other. Evolutionary biologists have used an episode from *Alice in Wonderland* by Lewis Caroll called the 'Red Queen' to describe this phenomenon.[3] The analogy is that in the same way as Alice and the Red Queen had to keep running just to stay in the same place, so viruses and their hosts have to keep evolving new attack and defence strategies in order for the virulence of the virus and the pathogenesis in the host to remain in balance.

With this in mind it is not surprising to find that in addition to specific immune mechanisms that provide antibodies and T cells to fight invading viruses, but which take some time to develop, more immediate defences are on hand. All primates produce 'host restriction factors', so called because they are molecules produced by cells to either prevent a virus from entering a cell or inhibit its

replication once inside. These factors have only recently been discovered, but already scientists have found a bewilderingly large
number of them ready and waiting inside cells to stall any potential invaders. They work through highly sophisticated and inter-
linked mechanisms, attacking all stages of the virus life cycle to
thwart virus genome replication and the production and release
of new virus particles. An expert has likened restriction factors to
HAART, the drug combination that keeps HIV infections at bay
by targeting the virus life cycle at several vital points.[4] One example is a family of restriction factors with an absurdly long name—
the 'apolipoprotein B editing complex catalytic subunits'. These
are cellular enzymes that inhibit retrovirus replication in a particularly ingenious way. Somehow they are packaged into new
virus particles as they assemble in an infected cell and so they are
carried on to the next cell that the viruses infect. Here they not
only suppress reverse transcription of the viral RNA into DNA
but also generate mutations in the virus genome that reduce its
ability to code for functional proteins.

Scientists interested in how genetic changes caused by our ancestors' experience of retrovirus infections might affect our susceptibility to HIV-1 have tracked the evolution of 140 genes thought to be in
some way implicated in HIV-1 infection and its pathogenesis. They
compared these gene sequences and those of 100 randomly chosen,
control genes in the genomes of five primate species (humans, chimpanzees, orang-utans (*Pongo pygmaeus*), rhesus monkey, and the
common marmoset (*Callithrix jacchus*)) that have been diverging
from each other for the past 40 million years or so. The scientists
came up with a list of thirteen genes, including several known
restriction factors, which have been positively selected in the human
genome. This means that compared to the control genes these

thirteen genes have an unexpectedly high level of mutations. This indicates rapid change in the proteins they code for, presumably driven by the need to counteract a series of new, lethal retrovirus infections encountered by our distant ancestors.[5] This is clear evidence that we have benefitted from our predecessors' experience with killer viruses by inheriting genes that code for proteins that give us some degree of protection. These proteins probably pose an insurmountable barrier to many potential invaders, but nevertheless we know that on occasions incoming SIVs have managed to sidestep restriction factors and set up persistent infections that cannot then be eliminated by more specific host immune mechanisms. This is the result of the fightback from retroviruses that have evolved ways and means of overcoming our battery of host defences.

The three main genes in a retrovirus genome, *gag*, *pol*, and *env*, are essential for virus infection and replication. In addition to these, all HIVs and most other primate lentiviruses have three or four extra genes, called accessory genes. These are not essential for virus replication in the laboratory but certainly affect the outcome of natural infection and transmission between hosts. The main function of the proteins coded by these genes, known as *vif* (virion infectivity factor), *vpr* (viral protein R), *vpu* (viral protein U) and *nef* (negative factor), is to allow the virus to infect, replicate, and spread inside a new host by neutralizing host defences. The fact that they have been conserved in most SIV genomes over millions of years of evolution indicates that they must form part of the viruses' essential survival kit. As details of their actions emerge it is becoming clear that they can explain some of the differences in pathogenesis between individual lentiviruses.

At present HIV-1 is the most pathogenic lentivirus known. An untreated HIV-1 infection increases the death rate up to sixty times, whereas at the other end of the scale, viruses like SIV_{smm} and SIV_{agm} do not affect the life expectancy of their respective hosts at all. HIV-2, the closest relative to SIV_{smm}, lies intermediate between these two extremes, increasing death rates in infected humans a modest two to five fold. We know from the work discussed in chapter 4 that SIV_{cpz}- infected chimpanzees living in Gombe National Park, Tanzania, show a ten to sixteen fold increase in mortality rate over uninfected animals, so placing SIV_{cpz} between HIV-1 and HIV-2 in the pathogenicity ranking. Although the reasons for this variable pathogenesis are not fully understood, it is noteworthy that those viruses that are relatively new to their hosts such as HIV-1 and HIV-2, as well as SIV_{cpz}, are more pathogenic than those like SIV_{smm} and SIV_{agm} that are thought to represent truly ancient infections. This is not surprising since these latter viruses have probably lived with their hosts over millions of years during which time they have co-evolved to maximize survival of both parties. But how has this been achieved?

As often happens, it was an astute clinical observation that pointed the way for scientific investigations into the pathogenicity of HIV-1. In 1995 Australian researchers described a group of seven HIV-1 positive people who had all been infected through infusion of contaminated blood or blood products from a single HIV-1 positive donor. All, including the donor, were long-term non-progressors, meaning that they were alive and well ten to fourteen years after initial infection with low or undetectable viral loads and normal CD4 T cell counts. Since the infecting virus was the only common factor linking them, scientists analysed viral genomes amplified from the blood of group members. They found that the group were all infected with a mutated virus with an absent *nef* gene but no other significant abnormalities.[6] A similar deletion in *nef* has been found in other HIV-1 long-term survivors, thus incriminating Nef (by convention the name of the protein coded for by *nef*) in determining the pathogenicity of the virus. These reports prompted further research into the functions of Nef in pathogenic and non-pathogenic SIVs.

In untreated HIV-1 infection it is the chronic loss of CD4 T cells that eventually causes immunodeficiency leading to fatal opportunistic infections. Immediately after primary HIV-1 infection large numbers of activated CD4 T cells appear in the blood, some of which are HIV-1 infected while others form part of the emerging immune response to the virus. All T cells that become activated for whatever reason die rapidly and estimates of T cell death during HIV-1 infection reach as high as a billion every day. This cycle of activation followed by cell death continues all through the silent, lag phase of HIV-1 infection, and although at first CD4 T cell numbers are maintained by increased production, eventually the capacity for replacement is exhausted. Then CD4 T cell numbers fall progressively and AIDS ensues. The average time between initial HIV-1 infection and development of AIDS is around ten years but this varies quite considerably between individuals. Clinicians find that the best predictors of progression to AIDS are the viral load and the proportion of CD4 T cells in the blood that are activated; the higher these are the more imminent the onset of AIDS. Thus it would seem logical to expect that these changes are not seen during infections with non-pathogenic retroviruses. In fact both SIV_{smm} and SIV_{agm} infections initially induce high levels of virus and activated CD4 T cells in the blood of their natural hosts. Critically though, while the viral load remains high, the number of activated CD4 T cells does not. The key to a non-pathogenic lentivirus infection is a reduction in the number of activated CD4 T cells after primary infection, thereby reducing T cell loss during the persistent infection. In this way a stable balance is achieved between T cell loss through infection and activation on the one hand and T cell renewal on the other. Thus, immunodeficiency is avoided and the infection remains non-pathogenic.

As it turns out it is the *nef* gene, present in all primate lentivirus virus genomes (excluding those few lucky long-term non-progressors infected with a mutant HIV-1), that has a major influence on T cell activation. Nef protein has evolved to counteract the immune response against viral proteins and this includes interfering with the function of CD4 T cells. The overall effect of Nef in non-pathogenic viruses like SIV_{smm} and SIV_{agm} is to reduce the expression of key host proteins involved in T cell activation, thereby preventing the lethal cycle of infection, activation, and T cell loss. Nef's function is highly conserved throughout primate lentivirus evolution and is no doubt essential for virus survival. By rendering the virus non-pathogenic it keeps the host alive, at the same time as allowing the virus to replicate sufficiently to spread to other hosts. Unfortunately though, the Nef proteins of SIV_{cpz} and all HIV-1 group viruses do not inhibit or reduce T cell activation, having lost the ability sometime during the evolution of SIV_{cpz} prior to its first jump to humans. We do not know exactly when or why this happened but it probably results from the rather complicated ancestry of HIV-1 uncovered by Sharp and his research group and outlined in chapter 3.

To recap, SIV_{cpz} is a recombinant virus made up of parts of the SIVs from the greater spot-nosed monkey (SIV_{gsn}) and the red-capped mangabey (SIV_{rcm}). Both of these viruses infected an individual *P.t.troglodytes* chimpanzee in which they subsequently recombined to form a new virus—SIV_{cpz}. This all took place a very long time ago, most likely before the split between *P.t.troglodytes* and *P.t.ellioti* subspecies. This would place it between 50,000 and 1M years ago, with the new virus subsequently spreading among chimpanzees ancestral to the subspecies *P.t.troglodytes* and *P.t.schweinfurthii*. It then jumped from the former to humans around 100 years ago. So far no one has studied Nef function in SIV_{rcm}, which provided the *nef* gene for SIV_{cpz}. However, its function must have been dispensed with somewhere along the line because SIV_{cpz} *vpu*, this time derived from SIV_{gsn}, now partly fulfil Nef's role by destroying CD4 molecules in infected cells. Nevertheless the overall result is that the balance is altered so that in HIV-1 and SIV_{cpz}, Nef actually enhances T cell activation and consequently all these viruses are pathogenic.[7]

A few inconsistencies in the Nef story indicate that it is not the only factor that controls the outcome of a lentivirus infection. Clearly lentiviruses that cause no disease in their natural hosts are not just non-pathogenic by nature. We know for instance that SIV_{smm} and SIV_{agm} can both cause simian AIDS in non-natural hosts; SIV_{smm} in rhesus macaques (SIV_{mac}, see chapter 2) and SIV_{agm} in pigtail macaques. Additionally, HIV-2, recently derived from SIV_{smm}, is pathogenic in humans, albeit to a lesser extent than HIV-1. Thus Nef, although important, cannot be the only determinant of pathogenicity. It is likely that it has other as yet unknown interactions with host proteins, and that unidentified host restriction factors as well as subtle differences in the immune response all compete to determine the outcome of a lentivirus infection.

Virus accessory genes are particularly important when a virus jumps from one host species to another because the alien environment in the new host's cells is likely to be extremely hostile. Indeed, most attempted host switches probably end in failure, yet the SIVs have quite a history of successful inter-species transmissions. As we know, ancestral HIV-1 alone has switched host several times in the fairly recent past, so perhaps it was the tiny accessory genes that facilitated this host-hopping. Scientists identified another restriction factor, called TRIM5α (one of the *tri*-partite *m*otif family of proteins), while trying to work out why rhesus macaques are resistant to HIV-1 infection. Originally they hoped that experimental infection of macaques would provide a model in which to study the pathogenesis of AIDS but this proved impossible because of rhesus TRIM5α. This protein binds to virus capsids as they enter a cell and destroys them. This aborts the infection before the viral genome has time to integrate into the host cell's DNA. However, not all lentivirus infections are blocked by all TRIM5α proteins. Primate TRIM5α proteins are among those that have evolved rapidly under pressure from ancient virus infections. Now they tend to only recognize the capsid proteins of lentiviruses that have infected their particular species. By replacing the capsid genes of HIV-1 with those from other lentiviruses experimentally, scientists worked out that in general TRIM5α proteins from higher primates, including chimpanzees and humans, can inhibit their own lentiviruses but not those from most monkey species.[8] Thus the inability of chimpanzee TRIM5α to inhibit incoming monkey lentiviruses must have facilitated colonization of the unfortunate *P.t.troglodytes* chimpanzee that sustained dual infection with SIV_{gsn} and SIV_{rcm}, which then recombined to form the ancestor of HIV-1.

Of course TRIM5α does not act alone to restrict lentivirus infections, but an interesting study on people at high risk of HIV-1 infection in Durban, South Africa, in 2009 suggests that it does have clinical relevance. Scientists found lower levels of TRIM5α expression in people infected with HIV-1 than in those without. Furthermore, they showed that the low TRIM5α expression levels were present before the HIV-1 infection and were not altered by it, indicating that the low levels were not induced by the virus infection itself.[9] Thus high expression of TRIM5α seems to reduce susceptibility to HIV-1 infection, a finding that may account for the relatively poor infectivity of the HIVs when compared to other sexually transmitted viruses (such as hepatitis B virus which is 300 times more infectious than HIV-1).

Perhaps the restriction factor that is most relevant to explaining the marked differences in epidemiology of HIV-1 group M, N, O and P viruses is tetherin, so called because it tethers virus particles to cell membranes. This cell protein prevents newly formed viruses inside one cell from spreading to others, a function that is not restricted to the HIVs as it has also been observed with Ebola viruses. Tetherin was discovered by scientists trying to find out why HIV-1 Vpu protein was necessary for the efficient release of virus particles from certain cell types but could be dispensed with in others. Ingeniously they fused these two cell types together experimentally to produce a hybrid cell, and then studied the outcome of its infection with HIV-1. As this always produced cells that required Vpu for virus particle release they deduced that they were chasing a factor present in the cells that normally prevented virus release and required Vpu to overcome this state. Eventually they succeeded in tracking it down.[10]

Tetherin sits in the cell membrane where it binds to and inactivates emerging viruses, that is, unless the virus has a way of stopping it. The fact that all SIVs have evolved ways of doing this suggests that the blocking effect of tetherin is an important hurdle for a virus to overcome when colonizing a new host. Some SIVs use their Vpu protein for this purpose (if they have one), but a few use Nef and some even employ their Env protein. Indeed, HIV-2 group A viruses use Env to counteract tetherin even though their immediate ancestor, SIV_{smm}, uses Nef in its natural host. At present we do not know whether HIV-2 groups B-H viruses have evolved a way of inhibiting human tetherin function but it would be interesting to find out. Any differences in this ability might explain why groups A and B have caused epidemics while the others struggled to survive in humans.

HIV-1, with several species switches in its fairly recent past, has an interesting record of parallel switching in tetherin-blocking devices. Its precursor, SIV_{cpz} gained its *vpu* gene from the greater spot-nosed monkey and its *nef* gene from the red-capped mangabey. It is most likely that SIV_{gsn} used Vpu to antagonize host tetherin just like its modern-day descendants. In contrast, we know that SIV_{rcm} must have used Nef because it does not have a *vpu* gene. Because chimpanzee and monkey tetherin molecules have diverged, it is unlikely that either protein functioned very efficiently after the viruses jumped to chimpanzees. In the event, it was the SIV_{rcm}-derived *nef* gene that evolved to block chimpanzee tetherin. Vpu from SIV_{gsn} then lost any tetherin blocking activity it might have had but retained the ability to destroy CD4 molecules. Thus when the recombinant SIV_{cpz} subsequently jumped to humans and gorillas it was Nef that had to interact with the new hosts' tetherin molecules. This worked fine in gorillas but not in humans. Compared to the chimpanzee tetherin gene the human equivalent has a small deletion that renders the protein insensitive to Nef from SIV_{cpz}. Just four amino acids are missing from the human protein, but since these are in the tail of the molecule, the very region that Nef binds to, Nef is inactive against it.

Thus in order to become established in humans SIV_{cpz} (and possibly SIV_{gor}) had to find an alternative way of counteracting tetherin. In the laboratory scientists can just replace the four amino acids missing from the tail of human tetherin to allow Nef to work, but this was not an option for incoming viruses. HIV-1 group M solved the problem by reverting to using Vpu like its distant ancestor, SIV_{gsn}, but this manoeuvre has not been so successful for HIV-1 groups O, N, and P viruses. Whereas in the laboratory Vpu from HIV-1 group M virus is a potent inhibitor of human tetherin, group O and P viruses are devoid of any such action. Vpu from group N viruses has a little anti-tetherin activity, but even this it appears to have been gained at the loss of another important function of Vpu, the destruction of CD4 molecules in infected cells.[11]

The tetherin protein interaction is the first adaptation discovered in HIV-1 that allows the virus to infect and replicate efficiently in human cells. And since it is more effective for HIV-1 group M than for groups N, O, and P viruses, it may also account for group M's remarkable propensity to spread. Certainly it is heralded as being a critical step in kickstarting the pandemic. When the findings were published in the scientific press the title of an accompanying review article held nothing back—A Tail of Tetherin: How Pandemic HIV-1 Conquered the World.[12]

* * *

The ongoing work on host restriction factors is at last revealing how HIV-1 group M could have outstripped all its competitors in its rapid and unrelenting spread around the world. Furthermore, in uncovering the biological and genetic differences between pathogenic and non-pathogenic viruses and their hosts, scientists are finding valuable clues to the pathogenesis of AIDS which are opening up new avenues for its prevention and treatment. In the final chapter we look at how the HIV-1 group M pandemic compares with past pandemics and discuss the lessons that can be learnt from it to help combat future killer viruses.

9

The Challenge of Pandemics

AIDS is the latest in a long list of fatal infectious diseases that have afflicted the human race. Well-known killers such as plague, smallpox, and Spanish flu have all, along with AIDS, caused pandemics that killed millions. Since the first description of AIDS in 1981 and the discovery of HIV in 1983, we have learnt a great deal about the history of both the disease and the virus, each new fact coming as a shock to experts and non-experts alike. In previous chapters we have traced HIV-1 group M's astonishing journey from its beginnings in west central Africa through to world dominance. We have uncovered where, when, how, and why the virus jumped to humans and how it subsequently spread internationally. In this concluding chapter we look back at pandemics experienced by our ancestors to see just how this modern scourge compares with the deadly plagues of the past. We then cast our gaze into the future to see how knowledge gained from unravelling the history of the HIVs can help in controlling their spread and preventing future pandemics.

Despite its limitations discussed in chapter 5, the molecular clock was indispensible in pinpointing the dates of the most recent common ancestors of the HIVs and SIVs, so providing vital clues for piecing together their ancient history and their present relationships. Equally, this ticking molecular metronome has been invaluable in uncovering the origin and history of many other epidemic and pandemic microbes. Like the HIVs, most 'new' human infectious diseases are *zoonoses*, meaning that they are caused by microbes that primarily infect animals but occasionally find a way of infecting humans. Over past millennia microbes have jumped from a surprisingly wide variety of both domestic and wild animals and proceeded to cause epidemics and pandemics. With the same molecular sequencing techniques, and evolutionary trees used to identify the origins of the HIVs, scientists have been able to uncover the origins of many of our ancient killers. The bacterium that causes bubonic plague, *Yersinia pestis*, for example, is primarily a rodent microbe that evolved as a blood parasite sometime within the last 20,000 years. It is spread within rodent communities by their fleas but, remarkably, it has never learnt to jump from one human to another. So even during pandemics each case of plague results from the bite of a rat flea that carries the deadly microbe. On the other hand, smallpox virus was an entirely human pathogen that spread from one victim to another through the air with relative ease. It had always been assumed that smallpox virus evolved from cowpox virus, the virus made famous by Edward Jenner after he used it to make the first ever vaccine. But evolutionary studies reveal its closest relatives to be the pox viruses of rodents and camels. Thus all three viruses must have arisen from a common ancestor, and the smallpox virus (*variola major*) probably first spread in humans in

Asia, possibly around 6,000 years ago.[1] Similarly, measles virus's closest relatives are rinderpest virus of cattle and to a lesser extent canine distemper virus. So again, all three viruses share a common ancestor, with measles and rinderpest viruses probably diverging around 2,000 years ago.[2]

Being inert particles, viruses have no say in where they go or who they infect. Their spread is all down to chance. But their ability to evolve rapidly allows them to exploit every available opportunity. The history of HIV-1 group M is punctuated by chance events without which the virus could not have flourished. Beginning with a jump between species, most probably resulting from an injury during a hunting trip, it was possibly then given the chance to adapt rapidly to its new host by contaminating unsterile injecting equipment. Travel from south east Cameroom to Kinshasa was the next chance event, and once there the virus laid low until its next big break came. The unique social mix in the city in the early 1900s, with its male predominance predisposing to epidemic levels of sexually transmitted diseases, gave the virus access to large sexual networks. Thus its exponential growth began. Even this could only have produced a few thousand infections by the early 1960s, but that was enough. When chance took the virus abroad its pandemic spread had begun.

Other historical occurrences just as disruptive as African colonialism in the 19th and early 20th centuries have allowed other microbes to emerge and become pandemic. In chapter 7 we have already seen how the European discovery of the Americas gave many Old World microbes the chance to reach the New World for the first time. Travelling along with slaves, traders, explorers, and immigrants they caused devastation. Smallpox and measles in particular, previously unknown in the Americas, wiped out whole tribes of Native Americans and thereby played a key role in the Spanish conquest of the Incas and Aztecs.

Perhaps the most spectacular social upheaval ever was the farming revolution which began around 11,000 years ago when our hunter-gatherer ancestors first domesticated plants and animals and settled down into farming communities. Literally hundreds of animal microbes took advantage of the new, close proximity to humans to colonize this new host. Emerging microbes of the day include the flu virus, which naturally infects wild birds. This virus could now use domestic water fowl as a stepping stone to infect humans and pigs, the latter often essential for adaptation before the virus could jump to humans.

Flu virus causes regular pandemics but none was as deadly as the 1918 Spanish flu. This new H1N1 strain of flu emerged just as the Great War was ending. It spread throughout the world in just six months, infecting 500 million—one-third of the world's population—and killing around 50 million people, many more than the estimated 10 million killed in the five years of combat. There is no doubt that the virus profited from the war with large troop encampments acting as breeding grounds and massive troop movements as dispersal agents. But why was it so deadly?

To answer this question scientists reconstructed a fossil flu virus genome preserved in the lungs of an Alaskan flu victim buried in the permafrost since 1918.[3] This revealed that all the viral genes came from an ancestral avian flu virus which had never before infected pigs or humans. Scientists then pinpointed the precise mutations that allowed the virus to infect and spread efficiently in humans and others that determined its virulence. Now these specific changes can be monitored in the H5N1 avian flu strain that is currently circulating in wild birds and has already

jumped to humans on several occasions. This is also a highly virulent virus but presently lacks the ability to spread between
humans. However, most flu experts think that it is only a matter
of time before this ability evolves. Hopefully, based on what we
have learnt from the 1918 flu strain, a vaccine can be prepared in
time to prevent its pandemic spread.

*　*　*

Epidemics and pandemics like plague, smallpox, measles, and flu
were clearly explosive, terrifying, and deadly. Caused by acute
infectious microbes, they spread rapidly and efficiently in
crowded, unhygienic living conditions. They then hitched a ride
with migrants, traders, armies, and travellers to disperse more
widely. With their short incubation periods, devastating illnesses,
and horrendously high death tolls, they could not be overlooked.
Even for people with no knowledge of microbes their infectious
nature was generally obvious, but not so HIV-1 group M. This
persistent virus causes no symptoms for many years, and so its
emergence passed unnoticed. This allowed it to spread widely
before it was recognized. However, even here there is a
precedent.

Transfer of microbes from primates to humans in sub-Saharan
Africa predates the farming revolution by several millennia. But as
living conditions among the sparse, mobile hunter-gatherer bands
populating Africa back then differed radically from those of farmers, so did the types of human microbes that emerged. Acute infectious microbes could not survive since, once everyone in a small
and isolated hunter gatherer band had been infected, their essential
chain of infection would be broken and they would die out. Only
those that establish persistent infections, so allowing the host to survive long enough to pass them on to their offspring, could maintain

a lifeline. Human T cell leukaemia virus is one such virus. Its closest relative is carried by several African primate species today and it is thought to have jumped to humans from a simian ancestor in central Africa on several occasions some tens of thousands of years ago. The virus has survived and diversified in humans ever since, reaching Japan, perhaps carried by traders as early as 300BC, and later arriving in the Caribbean via the slave trade (see chapter 7).

*   *   *

Clearly the one human activity that is key to microbe spread is our propensity to travel. And as our ancestors travelled further and further afield, so microbes followed along. Over the centuries they have benefitted from the step-wise collapse in travel time, well illustrated by the trip from the UK to Australia. This took a year in the 18th century, 100 days in the 19th and was reduced to 50 days by the introduction of steamships in the 20th. By the time SARS (severe acute respiratory syndrome) appeared at the beginning of the 21st century we could hop from any major city in the world to virtually any other within 24 hours. Planes are now airlifting over a billion people (holiday makers, businessmen, armies, pilgrims, refugees, migrants) to and from more than 200 countries every year.

One chance sneeze by a SARS coronavirus-infected doctor in a crowded elevator in an international hotel in Hong Kong disseminated the virus to twenty-seven different countries. No wonder alarm bells rang around the world. Fortunately though, because of the severe symptoms the virus causes and its inability to spread far through the air, SARS coronavirus was relatively easy to control. But not so HIV-1 group M. Just remember US patient zero who spread the virus in cities on two continents for several years while apparently in good health (see Figure 1, introduction).

*   *   *

Compared to flu, smallpox, plague, and SARS, HIV-1 group M's spread is remarkably slow and its infection rate is low. This is partly due to its sexual mode of transmission—very unusual for a pandemic microbe. The only other sexually transmitted disease that has become pandemic is syphilis caused by the bacterium *Treponema pallidum*. Its emergence in Spain at the end of the 15th century coincided with the return of Christopher Columbus and his crew from the Americas. In a reversal of the common flow of microbes at the time, it was assumed that the new disease had been brought from the New World by the explorers, but in fact even today the origin of syphilis is much debated. Nevertheless, the disease was first recognized in 1494 and rapidly spread throughout the whole of Europe, Asia, and North Africa. Like Spanish flu some 400 years later, the microbe's spread was aided by war. Its chance came when the French King, Charles VIII, raised an army and marched into Italy in an attempt to capture Naples. The new disease spread like wildfire among the troops, mercenaries, and camp followers. Charles himself was afflicted, and, perhaps as a result of this, he ordered a retreat. When the army disbanded, those who had picked up the microbe carried it back to their homelands where they sparked new epidemics. Syphilis has remained a common infection ever since, particularly in large cities like Paris, London, Berlin, and New York, where infection rates of 10–20 per cent were recorded until the advent of an effective treatment—penicillin—in the mid 20th century.

It is interesting that the finger pointing and blame reaction in the immediate wake of spreading syphilis was very similar to that caused by the emergence of AIDS six centuries later: 'The Italians called it the French disease, the French the disease of Naples, the Poles the German disease and the Russians the Polish disease. In the Middle East it was named the European pustule, in India the Franks, in China the ulcer of Canton, and in Japan Tang sore'.[4]

When syphilis arrived in Britain it was called 'the great pox' to distinguish it from the other common killer, smallpox. In today's terms this comparison seems misplaced but contemporary descriptions suggest that the symptoms of syphilis were far more severe then than they are today. Now *T pallidum* infection not only resembles HIV-1 in its mode of transmission but also in causing a relatively minor primary infection that could easily be overlooked. Both microbes persist in the body, but while virtually all those living with untreated HIV-1 eventually develop AIDS, only around a quarter of those with *T pallidum* develop tertiary syphilis with paralysis and dementia. And, importantly, while HIV-1 mainly targets young adults, syphilis generally remains silent until mid or late life. So while in global terms HIV-1's impact on society has been devastating, that of syphilis is restricted to the consequences on a few infected, influential rulers—possibly Ivan the Terrible of Russia and King Henry VIII of England.

* * *

Effective vaccines have been instrumental in abolishing pandemics of smallpox and measles, and have even facilitated the complete elimination of the former and the predicted demise of the latter. Where no vaccine is available, as in the case of syphilis, antimicrobial drugs can halt infection in an individual but cannot entirely prevent its spread to others. To date this is the case with HIV-1. Thirty years after its discovery and despite enormous expense and effort, we have HAART that prevents disease progression but no effective vaccine to interrupt its spread. The main reason for this has been uncovered by molecular and evolutionary biologists—the virus's rapid mutation rate that has generated such amazing genetic diversity. With all its subtypes and recombinant forms continuously evolving and diverging, vaccine production is an enormous challenge. Within one HIV-1 subtype, variation at the amino acid level reaches up to 30 per cent, while for measles virus, where a single vaccine is effective, this figure is around 4 per cent. Thus in reality a single vaccine is unlikely to prevent infection with all HIV-1 subtypes and variants. So how can molecular and evolutionary biologists help to design vaccines that can curtail the inexorable spread HIV-1 group M?

With their bank of thousands of HIV sequences accumulated over many years, perhaps scientists could identify genetic sequences common to clusters of virus subtypes and circulating recombinants. Then they could come up with a consensus amino acid sequence in the hope that it would induce immunity to the whole cluster of viruses. Alternatively, they could perhaps identify a vaccine candidate sequence in a virus ancestral to clusters of viruses that would induce broad immunity. To control flu virus, also a rapidly mutating RNA virus, a combination vaccine is prepared each year consisting of three currently circulating strains. Maybe a similar approach could be tried with HIV-1, using a different combination of vaccine strains to reflect the viruses circulating in particular geographical regions. Also similar to the work of scientists who reconstructed the 1918 flu virus, we have seen how HIV experts are beginning to hunt for mutations that relate to viral fitness. Again as this work progresses it should provide valuable information relating to vaccine preparation and drug design.

Many past pandemics continued for well over 100 years before they died out naturally. In modern times we expect to intervene to curtail the natural progression of pandemics, and indeed in thirty years we have come a long way in understanding and controlling HIV/AIDS. However, without a vaccine on the horizon to halt its progress, it is likely that the HIV pandemic will continue well into the 22nd century. In his address to the 18th International AIDS Conference in Vienna in 2010, former US President Bill Clinton, referring to recent successes in the fight against HIV/AIDS, paraphrased Sir Winston Churchill's famous speech given as the tide of World War II finally began to turn in Britain's favour: 'This is not the end. It's not even the beginning of the end. It is only the end of the beginning.'[5] With well over two million people still becoming infected with HIV-1 annually, those of us alive today will probably never know just how devastating the final outcome and global impact of the pandemic will be because we will not live to see it. But by understanding where, how, when, and why the virus evolved and spread among us, we can surely work to prevent the next one.

ENDNOTES

INTRODUCTION

1. Auerbach DM et al. *Am J Med* 76: 487–92. 1984.
2. <http://news.bbc.co.uk> 24 November 2003.
3. Pincock S. *Lancet* 372: 1373. 2008.
4. <http://history.nih.gov/nihinownwords/>. Accessed 15.12.2012.
5. <http://www.avert.org/aids-history-86.htm>. Accessed 15.12.2012.

1 THE PUZZLE OF HIV-1

1. Duesberg P and Ellison BJ. 1996. *Inventing the AIDS Virus*. Regnery Publishing Inc. Washington, US.
2. Chigwedere P et al. *J Acquir Immune Defic Syndr* 49: 410–15. 2008.
3. Duesberg P et al. *Med Hypotheses*. 19 July 2009.
4. <www.duesberg.com>. Accessed 15.12.12.
5. <www.duesberg.com>. Accessed 15.12.12.
6. Evans AS. *J Acquir Immune Defic Syndr* 2: 107–13. 1989.
7. Evans AS. *J Acquir Immune Defic Syndr* 2: 107–13. 1989.
8. CDC MMWR 31: 507–8, 513–14. 1982.
9. CDC MMWR 41: 961–2. 1993.
10. Duesberg P, Rasnick D. *Genetica* 104: 85–132. 1998.
11. Darby SC et al. *Nature* 377: 79–82. 1995.
12. Palca J. *Science* 256: 1130–1. 1992.
13. Cohen J. *Science* 266: 1647. 1994.
14. Chigwedere P and Essex M. *AIDS Behav* 14: 237–47. 2010.
15. Buonagurio DA et al. *Science* 232: 980–2. 1986.
16. Letvin NL et al. *PNAS* 80: 2718–22. 1983.
17. Henrickson RV et al. *Lancet* i: 388–90. 1983.
18. Mansfield KG et al. *J Med Primatol* 24: 116–22. 1995.
19. Daniel MD et al. *Science* 228: 1201–4. 1985.
20. Khan AS et al. *J Virol* 65: 7061–5. 1991.
21. Hirsch VM et al. *Nature* 339: 389–92. 1989.
22. Apetrei C et al. *J Virol* 79: 8991–9005. 2005.
23. Apetrei C et al. *AIDS* 20: 317–21. 2006.

24. Zigas V and Gajdusek DC. *Med J Australia* 2: 745–54. 1957.
25. Apetrei C et al. *J Virol* 79: 8991–9005. 2005.

2   TRACING HIV TO ITS ROOTS

1. Piot P et al. *Lancet* ii: 65–9. 1984.
2. Van de Perre P et al. *Lancet* ii: 62–5. 1984.
3. Serwadda D et al. *Lancet* ii: 849–52. 1985.
4. Berkley SF et al. *J Infect Dis* 160: 22–30. 1989.
5. Piot P et al. *J Infect Dis* 155: 1108–12. 1987.
6. Ronald AR et al. *Bull NY Acad Med* 64: 480–90. 1988.
7. Barin F et al. *Lancet* ii: 1387–9. 1985.
8. Clavel F et al. *Science* 233: 343–6. 1986.
9. Hirsch V et al. *Nature* 339: 389–92. 1989.
10. Chen Z et al. *J Virol* 70: 3617–26. 1996.
11. Wilkins A et al. *AIDS* 7: 1119–22. 1993.
12. Clavel F et al. *Science* 233: 343–6. 1986.
    Poulsen A-G et al. *Scand J Infect Dis* 32: 169–75. 2000.
13. Mota-Miranda A et al. *J Infect* 31: 163–4. 1995.
14. Lemey P et al. *PNAS* 100: 6588–92. 2003.
15. Santiago ML et al. *J Virol* 79: 12515–27. 2005.
16. Lemey P et al. *PNAS* 100: 6588–92. 2003.
17. For example: the *Sunday Express* 26 October 1986 'AIDS "made in lab" shock'. *The Sun* 3 January 1989 'Hitler created AIDS virus to destroy U.S.'.
18. Katner HP et al. *J Nat Med Ass* 79: 1068–72. 1987.
19. Huminer D et al. *Reviews of Infectious Diseases* 9: 1102–8. 1987.
20. Bygbjerg IC. *Lancet* i: 925. 1983.
21. Vandepitte J et al. *Lancet* i: 925–6. 1983.
22. Garry RF et al. *JAMA* 260: 2085–7. 1988.
23. Bayley AC. *Lancet* i: 1318–20. 1984.
24. Bayley AC et al. *Lancet* i: 359–61. 1985.
25. Williams G et al. *Lancet* ii: 951–5. 1960.
26. Corbitt G et al. *Lancet* 336: 51. 1990.
27. Frøland SS et al. *Lancet* i 1344–5. 1988.
28. Nzilambi N et al. *N Engl J Med* 318: 276–9. 1988.
29. Nahmias AJ et al. *Lancet* i: 1279–80. 1986.
30. De Leys R et al. *J Virol* 64: 1207–16. 1990.
31. Simon F et al. *Nature Medicine* 4: 1032–7. 1998.
32. Jonassen TO. *Virology*: 234: 43–7. 1997.
33. Vidal N et al. *J Virol* 74: 10498–507. 2000.

34. Zhu T and Ho DD. *Nature* 374: 503–4. 1995.
35. Zhu T et al. *Nature* 391: 594–7. 1998.

3   THE PRIMATE CONNECTION

1. Sharp PM et al. *Phil Trans R Soc Lond B* 349:41–7. 1995.
2. Jin MJ et al. *J Virol* 68: 8454–60. 1994.
3. Jin MJ et al. *EMBO* 13: 2935–47. 1994.
4. Peeters M et al. *AIDS* 3: 625–30. 1989.
5. Peeters M et al. *AIDS* 6: 447–51. 1992.
6. Gilden RV et al. *Lancet* i: 678–9. 1986.
7. Morin PA et al. *Science* 265:1193–201. 1994.
8. Gonder MK et al. *Nature* 388: 337. 1997.
9. Gao F et al. *Nature* 397: 436–8. 1999.
10. Bailes E et al. *Science* 300: 1713. 2003.

4   FROM RAINFOREST TO RESEARCH LABORATORY

1. Corbet S et al. *J Virol* 74: 529–34. 2000.
2. Leroy EM et al. *Science* 303: 387–90. 2004.
3. Santiago ML et al. *Science* 295: 465. 2002.
4. Keele BF et al. *Science* 313: 523–6. 2006.
5. Van Heuverswyn F et al. *Nature* 444: 164. 2006.
6. Takehisa J et al. *J Virol* 83: 1635–48. 2009.
7. Takehisa J et al. *Journal of Virology* 83: 1635–48. 2009.
8. Neel C et al. *J Virol* 84: 1464–76. 2010.
9. Plantier J-C et al. *Nature Medicine* 15: 871–2. 2009.
10. Vallari A et al. *J Virol* 85: 1403–7. 2011.
11. Keele BF et al. *Nature* 460: 515–19. 2009.
12. Rudicell RS et al. *PloS Pathogens* 6: e1001116. 2010.
13. Etienne L et al. *Retrovirol* 8: 4. 2011.

5   TIMING THE JUMP

1. Zhu et al. *Nature* 391: 594–7. 1998.
2. Smith TF et al. *Nature* 333: 573–5. 1988.
3. Mulder C. *Nature* 333: 396. 1988.
4. Li W-H et al. *Mol Biol Evol* 5: 313–30. 1988.
5. Korber B et al. *Science* 280: 1868. 1998.
6. Sharp PM et al. *Biochem Soc Trans* 28: 275–82. 2000.

7. Korber B et al. *Science* 288: 1789–96. 2000.
8. Salemi M et al. *FASEB J* 15: 276–8. 2001.
9. Worobey M et al. *Science* 329: p. 1487. 2010.
10. Li W-H et al. *Mol Biol Evol* 5: 313–30. 1988.
11. Robertson DL et al. *Nature* 374: 124–6. 1995.
12. Wolinsky SM et al. *Science* 272:537–42. 1996.
13. Smith DG. *Lancet* 335: 781–2. 1990.
14. Yusim K et al. *Phil Trans R Soc Lond* B 3566:855–66. 2001.
15. Leitner T et al. *PNAS* 93: 10864–9. 1996.
16. Leitner T et al. *PNAS* 96: 10752–7. 1999.
17. Worobey M et al. *Nature* 455: 661–4. 2008.
18. Pitchenik AE et al. *Annals of Int Med* 98: 277–84. 1983.
19. Pape JW et al. *New Engl J Med* 309: 945–50. 1983.
20. Li W-H et al. *Mol Biol Evol* 5: 313–30. 1988.
21. Gilbert MTP et al. *PNAS* 104:1856–70. 2007.
22. Cohen J. *Science* 318: 731. 2007.

6 VITAL FIRST STEPS

1. Gilks C. *Nature* 354: 262. 1991.
2. Kuvin SF. *Nature* 355: 305. 1992.
3. Curtis T. *Rolling Stone* 626: 54–60. 1992.
4. Courtois G et al. *BMJ* 26 July 187–109. 1958.
5. Li W-H et al. *Mol Biol Evol* 5: 313–30. 1988.
6. Martin B. *J Med Ethics* 29: 253–6. 2003.
7. Hooper E. *The River: A journey to the source of HIV and AIDS*. Back Bay Books, Little, Brown and Company, Boston, New York, London. 1999.
8. Hooper E. *The River: A journey to the source of HIV and AIDS*. Back Bay Books, Little, Brown and Company, Boston, New York, London. p. xxviii. 1999.
9. Basilico C et al. *Report from the AIDS/Polio Advisory Committee*. 18 September 1992.
10. Zhu T and Ho DD. *Nature* 374: 503–4. 1995.
11. Hooper E. *Phil Trans R Soc Lond* B 356, 803–14. 2001.
12. Hooper E. *Phil Trans R Soc Lond* B 356, 803–14. 2001.
13. Hooper E. *Phil Trans R Soc Lond* B 356, 803–14. 2001.
14. Dawkins R. *The Selfish Gene*. Oxford University Press, Oxford. 1976.
15. May RM *Phil Trans R Soc Lond* B 356, 785–787. 2001.

16. Trivers R. *Nature* 404: 828. 2000.
17. Grafen A. *Biogr Mem Fell R Soc Lond* 50: 109–32. 2004.
18. *Phil Trans R Soc Lond B* 356. 2001.
19. Basilico C et al. *Report from the AIDS/Polio Advisory Committee*. 18 September 1992.
20. *Phil Trans R Soc Lond B* 356, 947–53. 2001.
21. <www.aidsorigins.com> Accessed 15.12.2012. <www.bmartin.co.uk/>. Website returning soon.
22. Medawar PB. *Advice to a young scientist*. Basic Books. Perseus Books group. p 39. 1979.
23. Weiss RA. *Nature* 410: 1035–6. 2001.
24. Vidal N et al. *J Virol* 74:10498–507. 2000.
25. Rambaut A et al. *Nature* 410: 1047–8. 2001.
26. Worobey M et al. *Nature* 428: 820. 2004.

7   THE EPIC JOURNEY BEGINS

1. Chitnis A et al. *AIDS Res Hum Retroviruses* 16: 5–8. 2000.
2. Meiering CD and Linial ML. *Clin Microbiol Reviews* 14: 165–76. 2001.
3. Wolfe ND et al. *Lancet* 363: 932–7. 2004.
4. Peeters M et al. *Emerg Infect Dis* 8: 451–7. 2002.
5. Souquiere S et al. *J Virol* 75: 7086–96. 2001.
6. Kalish ML et al. *Emerg Infect Dis* 11: 1928–30. 2005.
7. Pépin J. *The origin of AIDS*. Cambridge University Press, Cambridge. p. 60. 2011.
8. Joag et al. *J Virol* 70: 3189–97. 1996.
9. Marx PA et al. *Phil Trans R Soc Lond B* 356: 911–20. 2001.
10. Drucker E et al. *Lancet* 358: 1989–92. 2001.
11. Frank C et al. *Lancet* 355: 887–91. 2000.
12. Frank C et al. *Lancet* 355: 887–91. 2000.
13. Pépin J et al. *CID* 51: 768–76. 2010.
14. Pépin J et al. *CID* 51: 777–84. 2010.
15. Worobey M et al. *Nature* 455: 661–4. 2008.
16. Niama FR et al. *Infect Genet Evol* 6: 337–43. 2006.
17. Hayes RJ et al. *J Trop Med Hyg* 98: 1–8. 1995.
18. Cameron DW et al. *Lancet* ii: 403–7. 1989.
19. Sousa JD et al. *PLoS ONE* 5: e9936. 2010.
20. Sousa JD et al. *PLoS ONE* 5: e9936. 2010.

8 ADAPTING TO HUMANS

1. Arien KK et al. *Nature Rev Microbiol* 5: 141–51. 2007.
2. Wain LV et al. *Mol Biol Evol* 24: 1853–60. 2007.
3. Van Valen L. *Evol Theory* 1:1–30. 1973.
4. Kirchhoff F. *Cell Host & Microbe* 8: 55–67. 2010.
5. Ortiz M et al. *Mol Biol Evol* 26: 2865–75. 2009.
6. Deacon NJ et al. *Science* 270: 988–91. 1995.
7. Schlinder M et al. *Cell* 125: 1055–67. 2006.
8. Kratovac Z et al. *J Virol* 82: 6772–7. 2008.
9. Sewram S et al. *JID* 199: 1657–63. 2009.
10. Neil SJ et al. *Nature* 451: 425–31. 2008.
11. Sauter D et al. *Cell Host & Microbe* 6: 409–21. 2009.
12. Gupta RK and Towers GJ. *Cell Host & Microbe* 6: 393–5. 2009.

9 THE CHALLENGE OF PANDEMICS

1. Li Y et al. *PNAS* 104: 15787–92. 2007.
2. Furuse Y et al. *Virology Journal* 7: 52. 2010.
3. Taubenberger JK et al. *Nature* 437: 889–93. 2005.
4. Crawford DH. Deadly Companions: How microbes shaped world history. Oxford University Press, Oxford. 2007.
5. <http://www.voanews.com/content/decapua-aids2010-bill-clinton-19jul10-98751964/155386.html>. Accessed 15.12.2012.

REFERENCES

'AIDSOrigins', <www.aidsorigins.com>. Edward Hooper's site on the origins of AIDS.

Apetrei C., Kaur, A., Lerche, N., Metzger, M., Pandrea, I., Hardcastle, J., Falkenstein, S., Bohm, R., Koehler, J., Traina-Dorge, V., Williams, T., Straprans, S., Plauche, G., Veazey, R. S., McClure, H., Lackner, A. A., Gormus, B., Robertson, D., L., and Marx, P. A. (2005), 'Molecular epidemiology of simian immunodeficiency virus SIVsm in U.S. primate centers unravels the origin of SIVmac and SIVstm', *Journal of Virology* 79: 8991–9005.

Apetrei C., Lerche, N. W., Pandrea, I., Gormus, B., Silvestri, G., Kaur, A., Robertson, D.L., Hardcastle, J., Lackner, A. A., and Marx, P. A. (2006), 'Kuru experiments triggered the emergence of pathogenic SIVmac', *AIDS* 20: 317–21.

Arien, K. K., Vanham, G., and Arts, E. J. (2007), 'Is HIV-1 evolving to a less virulent form in humans?' *Nature Reviews Microbiology* 5: 141–51.

Auerbach D. M., Darrow W. W., Jaffe H. W., and Curran J. W. (1984), 'Cluster of cases of the acquired immune deficiency syndrome. Patients linked by sexual contact', *American Journal of Medicine* 76: 487–92.

Avert 'History of AIDS Up to 1986'. Available at <http://www.avert.org/aids-history-86.htm>.

Bailes E., Gao, F., Bibollet-Ruche, F., Courgnaud, V., Peeters, M., Marx, P. A., Hahn, B. H., and Sharp, P. M. (2003), 'Hybrid origin of SIV in chimpanzees', *Science* 300: 1713.

Barin, F., M'Boup, S., Denis, F., Kanki, P., Allan, J. S., Lee, T. H., and Essex, M. (1985), 'Serological evidence for virus related to simian T-lymphotropic retrovirus III in residents of west Africa,' *The Lancet* ii: 1387–9.

Basilico, C., Buck, C., Desrosiers, R., Ho, D., Lilly, F., and Wimmer, E. (1992), *Report from the AIDS/Poliovirus Advisory Committee*, 18 September.

Bayley, A. C. (1984), 'Aggressive Kaposi's sarcoma in Zambia', *The Lancet* 1: 1318–20.

Bayley, A. C., Downing, R. G., Cheingsong-Popov, R., Tedder, R. S., Dalgleish, A. G., and Weiss, R. A. (1985), 'HTLV-III serology distinguishes atypical and endemic Kaposi's sarcoma in Africa', *The Lancet* i: 359–61.

Berkley, S. F., Widywirski, R., Okware, S. I., Downing, R., Linnan, M. J., White, K. E., et al. (1989), 'Risk-factors associated with HIV infection in Uganda', *Journal of Infectious Diseases*, 160(1), 22–30.

Buonagurio, D. A., Nakada, S. S., Parvin, J. D., Krystal, M. M., Palese, P. P., and Fitch, W. M. (1986), 'Evolution of human influenza A viruses over 50 years: Rapid, uniform rate of change in NS gene', *Science* 232: 980–2.

Bygbjerg, I. C. (1983), 'AIDS in a Danish surgeon (Zaire, 1976)', *The Lancet* i: 925. 1983.

Cameron, D. W., Simonsen, J. N., D'Costa, L. J., Ronald, A. R., Maitha, G. M., Gakinya, M. N., Cheang, M., Ndinya-Achola, J. O., Piot, P., Brunham, R. C., et al. (1989), 'Female to male transmission of human immunodeficiency virus type 1: Risk factors for seroconversion in men', *The Lancet* ii: 403–7.

Chen, Z., Telfier, P., Gettie, A., Reed, P., Zhang, L., Ho, D. D., and Marx, P. A. (1996), 'Genetic characterization of new West African simian immunodeficiency virus SIVsm: geographic clustering of household-derived SIV strains with human immunodeficiency virus type 2 subtypes and genetically diverse viruses from a single feral sooty mangabey troop', *Journal of Virology* 70: 3617–26.

Chigwedere, P, and Essex, M. (April 2010), 'AIDS denialism and public health practice', *AIDS and Behavior* 14: 237–47.

Chigwedere, P., Seage, G., Gruskin, S., Lee, T., and Essex, M. (2008), 'Estimating the lost benefits of antiretroviral drug use in South Africa', *Journal of Acquired Immune Deficiency Syndrome* 49: 410–5.

Chitnis, A., Rawls, D., and Moore, J. (2000). 'Origin of HIV Type 1 in Colonial French Equatorial Africa?' *AIDS Research and Human Retroviruses* 16: 5–8.

Clavel, F., Guetard, D., Brun-Vezinet, F., et al. (1986), 'Isolation of a new human retrovirus from West African patients with AIDS', *Science* 233: 343–6.

Clinton, W. J., *Voice of America*, 'Bill Clinton on HIV/AIDS: Much More Needs to be Done'. Available at <http://www.voanews.com/content/decapua-aids2010-bill-clinton-19jul10-98751964/155386.html>.

Cohen J. (1994), 'Could drugs rather than a virus be the cause of AIDS?' *Science* 266: 1647.

Cohen Y., (2007) 'Reconstructing the origins of the AIDS epidemic from archived HIV isolates', *AIDS Research*, 318: 731.

Corbet, S., Muller-Trutwin, M. C., Versmisse, P., Delarue, S., Ayouba, A., Lewis, J,. Brunak, S., Martin, P., Brun-Vezinet, F., Simon, F., Barre-Sinoussi, F., and Mauclere, P. (2000), '*Env* sequences of simian immunodeficiency viruses from chimpanzees in Cameroon are strongly related to those of human immunodeficiency virus group N from the same geographic area', *Journal of Virology* 74: 529–34.

Corbitt, G., Bailey, A. S., and Williams, G. (1990), 'HIV infection in Manchester, 1959', *The Lancet* 336: 51.

Courtois, G., Flack, A., Jervis, G. A., Koprowski, H., and Ninane, G. (1958), 'Preliminary report on mass vaccination of man with live attenuated poliomyelitis virus in the Belgian Congo and Ruanda-Urundi', *British Medical Journal*, 2: 187–190.

Crawford D. H. (2007), *Deadly Companions: How microbes shaped world history*. Oxford: Oxford University Press.

Curtis T. (1992), 'The Origin of Aids', *Rolling Stone* 626: 54–60.

Daniel, M. D., Letvin, N. L., King, N. W., Kannagi, M., Sehgal, P. K., Hunt, R. D., Kanki, P. J., Essex, M., and Desrosiers, R. C. (1985), 'Isolation of T-cell tropic HTLV-III-like retrovirus from macaques', *Science* 228: 1201–4.

Darby, S. C., Ewart, D. W., Giangrande, P. L., Dolin, P. J, Spooner, R. J., and Rizza, C. R. (1995), 'Mortality before and after HIV infection in the complete UK population of haemophiliacs', *Nature* 377: 79–82.

Dawkins, R. (1976), *The Selfish Gene*. Oxford: Oxford University Press.

Deacon, N. J., Tsykin, A., Solomon, A., Smith, K., Ludford-Menting, M., Hooker, D. J., McPhee, D. A., Greenway, A. L., Ellett, A., Chatfield, C., Lawson, V. A., Crowe, S., Maerz, A., Sonza S., Learmont, J., Sullivan, J. S., Cunningham, A., Dwyer, D., Dowton, D., and Mills, J. (1995), 'Genomic structure of an attenuated quasi species of HIV-1 from a blood transfusion donor and recipients', *Science* 270: 988–91.

De Leys, R., Vanderborght, B., Vanden Haesevelde, M., Heyndrickx, L., van Geel, A., Wauters, C., Bernaerts, R., Saman, E., Nijs, P., Willems, B., et al. (1990), 'Isolation and partial characterization of an unusual human immunodeficiency retrovirus from two persons of west-central African origin', *Journal of Virology* 64: 1207–16.

Drucker, E., Alcabes, P. G., and Marx, P. A. (2001), 'The injection century: Massive unsterile injections and the emergence of human pathogens', *The Lancet* 358: 1989–92.

Duesberg on Aids [website] <www.duesberg.com>.

Duesberg, P. H., and Ellison, B. J. (1996), *Inventing the AIDS Virus*. Washington, US: Regnery Publishing Inc.

Duesberg, P. H., Nicholson, J. M., Rasnick, D., Fiala, C., and Bauer, H. H. (July 2009). 'HIV-AIDS hypothesis out of touch with South African AIDS: A new perspective', *Medical Hypotheses*.

Duesberg, P. H. and Rasnick, D. (1998), 'The AIDS dilemma: Drug diseases blamed on a passenger virus', *Genetica* 104: 85–132.

Etienne, L., Nerrienet, E., LeBreton, M., Bibila, G. T., Foupouapouognigni, Y., Rousset, D., Nana, A., Djoko, C. F., Tamoufe, U., Aghokeng, A. F., et al. (2011), 'Characterization of a new simian immunodeficiency virus strain in a naturally infected Pan troglodytes troglodytes chimpanzee with AIDS related symptoms', *Retrovirology* 8: 4.

Evans A. S. (1989), 'Does HIV cause AIDS? An historical perspective', *Journal of Acquired Immune Deficiency Syndromes* 2: 107–13.

Frank, C., Mohamed, M. K., Strickland, G. T., Lavanchy, D., Arthur, R. R., Magder, L. S., El Khoby, T., Abdel-Wahab, Y., Aly Ohn, E. S., Anwar, W., and Sallam, I. (2000), 'The role of parenteral antischistosomal therapy in the spread of hepatitis C virus in Egypt', *The Lancet* 355: 887–91.

Frøland, S. S., Jenum, P., Lindboe, C. F., Wefring, K. W., Linnestad, P. J., and Böhmer, T. (1988) 'HIV-1 infection in Norwegian family before 1970'.

Furuse, Y., Suzuki, A., and Oshitani, H. (2010), 'Origin of measles virus: Divergence from rinderpest virus between the 11th and 12th centuries', *Virology Journal* 7: 52.

Gao, F., Robertson, D. L., Carruthers, C. D., et al. (1999), 'Origin of HIV-1 in the chimpanzee *Pan troglodytes troglodytes*', *Nature* 397: 436–441.

Garry, R. F., Witte, M. H., Gottleib, A. A., et al (1988), 'Documentation of an AIDS virus infection in the United States in 1968', *JAMA* 260: 2085–2087.

Gilbert, M. T., Rambaut, A., Wlasiuk, G,, Spira, T. J., Pitchenik, A. E., Worobey, M., et al. (2007), 'The emergence of HIV/AIDS in the Americas and beyond', *PNAS* 104:1856–70.

Gilden, R. V., Arthur, L. O., Robey, W. G., et al. (1986), 'HTLV-III antibody in a breeding chimpanzee not experimentally exposed to the virus.' *The Lancet* i: 678–679.

Gilks C. (1991), 'AIDS, monkeys, and malaria', *Nature* 354: 262. 1991

Gonder, M. K., Oates, J. F., Disotell, T. R., Forstner, M. R., Morales, J. C., et al. (1997), 'A new west African chimpanzee subspecies?' *Nature* 388: 337.

Grafen, A. (2004), 'William Donald Hamilton 1 August 1936–7 March 2000', *Biographical Memoirs of Fellows of the Royal Society London* 50: 109–32.

Gupta, R. K. and Towers G. J. (2009), 'A tail of Tetherin: How pandemic HIV-1 conquered the world', *Cell Host & Microbe* 6: 393–5.

Hayes, R. J., Schulz, K., and Plummer, F. A. (1995), 'The cofactor effect of genital ulcers on the per-exposure risk of HIV transmission in sub-Saharan Africa', *Journal of Tropical Medicine and Hygiene.* 98: 1–8.

Henrickson R. V., Maul, D. H., Osborn, K. G., Sever, J. L., Madden, D. L., Ellingsworth, L. R., Anderson, J. H., Lowenstine, L. J., and Gardner, M. B. (1983), 'Epidemic of acquired immunodeficiency in rhesus monkeys', *The Lancet* i: 388–390.

Hirsch V. M., Olmsted R. A., Murphey-Corb, M., Purcell, R. H., and Johnson, P. R. (1989), 'An African primate lentivirus (SIVsm) closely related to HIV-2', *Nature* 339: 389–92.

Hooper, E. (1999), *The River: A journey to the source of HIV and AIDS.* Boston, New York, London: Back Bay Books, Little, Brown and Company.

Hooper, E. (2001), 'Experimental oral polio vaccines and acquired immune deficiency syndrome', *Philosophical Transactions of the Royal Society London B* 356: 803–14.

Huminer D., Rosenfeld, J. B., and Pitlik, S. D. (1987), 'AIDS in the pre-AIDS era', *Reviews of Infectious Diseases* 9: 1102–8.

In Their Own Words [website] <http://history.nih.gov/nihinownwords>.

Jin, M. J., Rogers, J., Phillips-Conroy, J. E., Allan, J. S., Desrosiers, R. C., Shaw, G. M., Sharp, P. M., and Hahn, B. H. (1994), 'Infection of a yellow baboon with simian immunodeficiency virus from African green monkeys: Evidence for cross-species transmission in the wild', *Journal of Virology.* 68: 8454–60.

Jin, M. J., Hui, H., Robertson, D. L., et al. (1994), 'Mosaic genome structure of simian immunodeficiency virus from West African green monkeys', *The EMBO Journal* 13: 2935–47.

Joag, S. V., Li, Z., Wang, C., Jia, F., Foresman, L., Adany, I., Pinson, D. M., Stephens, E. B., and Narayan, O. (1996), 'Chimeric SHIV that causes CD4+ T cell loss and AIDS in rhesus macaques', *Journal of Virology*. 70: 3189–97.

Jonassen, T. O. (1997), 'Sequence analysis of HIV-1 group O from Norwegian patients infected in the 1960s', *Virology*: 234: 43–7.

Kalish M. L., Wolfe, N. D., Ndongmo, C. B., McNicholl, J., Robbins, K. E., Aidoo, M. et al. (2005), 'Central African hunters exposed to simian immunodeficiency virus', *Emerging Infectious Diseases* 11: 1928–30.

Katner, H. P. and Pankey, G. A. (1987), 'Evidence for a Euro-American origin of human immunodeficiency virus (HIV)', *Journal of the National Medical Association* 79: 1068–72.

Keele, B. F., Van Heuverswyn, F., Li, Y., Bailes, E., Takehisa, J., Santiago, M. L., Bibollet-Ruche, F., Chen, Y., Wain, L. V., Liegeois, F., Loul, S., Ngole, E. M., Bienvenue, Y., Delaporte, E., Brookfield, J. F., Sharp, P. M., Shaw, G. M., Peeters, M., and Hahn, B. H. (2006), 'Chimpanzee reservoirs of pandemic and nonpandemic HIV-1', *Science* 313: 523–6.

Keele, B. F., Jones, J. H., Terio, K. A., Estes, J. D., Rudicell, R. S., Wilson, M. L., Li, Y., Learn, G. H., Beasley. T. M., Schumacher-Stankey, J., Wroblewski, E., Mosser, A., Raphael, J., Kamenya, S., Lonsdorf, E. V., Travis, D. A., Mlengeya, T., Kinsel, M. J., Else, J. G., Silvestri, G., Goodall, J., Sharp, P. M., Shaw, G. M., Pusey, A. E., and Hahn, B. H. (2009), 'Increased mortality and AIDS-like immunopathology in wild chimpanzees infected with SIVcpz', *Nature* 460: 515–19.

Khan, A. S., Galvin, T. A., Lowenstine, L. J., Jennings, M. B., Gardner, M. B., and Buckler, C. E. (1991), 'A highly divergent simian immunodeficiency virus (SIVstm) recovered from stored stump-tailed macaque tissues', *Journal of Virology* 65: 7061–5.

Kirchhoff, F. (2010), 'Immune evasion and counteraction of restriction factors by HIV-1 and other primate lentiviruses', *Cell Host & Microbe* 8: 55–67.

Korber, B., Theiler, J., and Wolinsky, S. (1998), 'Limitations of a molecular clock applied to considerations of the origin of HIV-1', *Science* 280: 1868.

Korber, B., Muldoon, M., Theiler, J., Gao, F., Gupta, R., Lapedes, A., Hahn, B. H., Wolinsky, S., and Bhattacharya, T. (2000), 'Timing the ancestor of the HIV-1 pandemic strains', *Science* 288: 1789–96.

Kratovac, Z., Virgen, C. A., Bibollet-Ruche, F., Hahn, B. H., Bieniasz, P. D., and Hatziioannou, T. (2008), 'Primate lentivirus capsid sensitivity to TRIM5 proteins', *Journal of Virology* 82: 6772–7.

Kuvin, S. F. (1992), 'AIDS and malaria experiments', *Nature* 355: 305.

Leitner, T., Escanilla, D., Franzen, C., et al. (1996) 'Accurate reconstruction of a known HIV-1 transmission history by phylogenetic tree analysis', *PNAS* 93: 10864–9.

Leitner, T. and Albert, J. (1999), 'The molecular clock of HIV-1 unveiled through analysis of a known transmission history', *PNAS* 96: 10752–7.

Lemey, P., Pybus, O. G., Wang, B., Saksena, N. K., Salemi, M., and Vandamme, A. M. (2003), 'Tracing the origin and history of the HIV-2 epidemic', *PNAS* 100: 6588–92.

Leroy, E. M., Rouquet, P., Formenty, P., Souquière, S., Kilbourne, A., Froment, J. M., Bermejo, M., Smit, S., Karesh, W., Swanepoel, R., Zaki, S. R., and Rollin, P. E. (2004), 'Multiple Ebola virus transmission events and rapid decline of central African wildlife', *Science* 303:387–390.

Letvin, N. L., Daniel, M. D., Sehgal, P. K., Chalifoux, L. V. King, N. W., Hunt, R. D., Aldrich, W. R., Holley, K., Schmidt, D. K., and Desrosiers, R. C. (1983), 'Experimental infection of rhesus monkeys with type D retrovirus', *PNAS* 80: 2718–22.

Li, W.-H., Tanimura, M., and Sharp, P. M. (1988), 'Rates and dates of divergence between AIDS virus nucleotide sequences', *Molecular Biology and Evolution* 5: 313–30.

Li, Y., Carroll, D. S., Gardner, S. N., Walsh, M. C., Vitalis, E. A., and Damon, I. K. (2007), 'On the origin of smallpox: Correlating variola phylogenics with historical smallpox records', *PNAS* 104: 15787–92.

Mansfield, K. G., Lerche, N. W., Gardner, M. B., and Lacker, A. A. (1995), 'Origins of simian immunodeficiency virus infection in macaques at the New England Regional Primate Research Center', *Journal of Medical Primatology* 24: 116–22.

Martin, B. (2003), 'Investigating the origin of AIDS: Some ethical dimensions', *Journal of Medical Ethics* 29: 253–6.

Marx, P. A., Alcabes, P. G., and Drucker, E. (2001), 'Serial human passage of simian immunodeficiency virus by unsterile injections and the emergence of epidemic human immunodeficiency virus in Africa', *Philosophical Transactions of the Royal Society London B* 356: 911–20.

May, R. M. (2001), 'Memorial to Bill Hamilton', *Philosophical Transactions of the Royal Society London B* 365: 785–787.

Medawar P. B. (1979), *Advice to a young scientist*. New York: Basic Books, Perseus Books Group.

Meiering, C. D. and Linial, M. L. (2001), 'Historical perspective of foamy virus epidemiology and infection', *Clinical Microbiology Reviews* 14: 165–76.

Morin, P. A., Moore, J. J., Chakraborty, R., Jin, L., Goodall, J., and Woodruff, D. S. (1994), 'Kin selection, social structure, gene flow, and the evolution of chimpanzees', *Science* 265: 1193–1201.

Mota-Miranda, A., Gomes, H., Marques, R., Serrão, R., Lourenç, O. H., Santos Ferreira, O., and Lecour, H. (1995), 'HIV-2 infection with a long asymptomatic period—a case report', *Journal of Infection* 31: 163–4.

Mulder, C. (1988), 'Human AIDS virus not from monkeys', *Nature* 333: 396.

Nahmias, A. J., Weiss, J., Yao, X., Lee, F., Kodsi, R., Schanfield, M., Matthews, T., Bolognesi, D., Durack, D., Motulsky, A., et al. (1986), 'Evidence for human infection with an HTLV III/LAV-like virus in Central Africa, 1959', *The Lancet.* i:1279–1280.

Neel, C., Etienne, L., Li, Y., et al. (2010), 'Molecular epidemiology of simian immunodeficiency virus infection in wild-living gorillas', *Journal of Virology*, 84, 1464–76.

Neil, S. J., Zang, T., and Bieniasz, P. D. (2008), 'Tetherin inhibits retrovirus release and is antagonized by HIV-1 Vpu', *Nature* 451: 425–31.

Niama, F. R., Toure-Kane, C., Vidal, N., et al. (2006), 'HIV-1 subtypes and recombinants in the Republic of Congo', *Infection, Genetics and Evolution* 6: 337–343.

Nzilambi, N., De Cock, K. M., Forthal, D. N., et al. (1988), 'The prevalence of infection with human immunodeficiency virus over a 10-year period in rural Zaire', *New England Journal of Medicine* 318: 276–9.

Ortiz, M., Guex, N., Patin, E., Martin, O., Xenarios, I., Ciuffi, A., Quintana-Murci, L., and Telenti, A. (2009), 'Evolutionary trajectories of primate genes involved in HIV pathogenesis', *Molecular Biology and Evolution* 26: 2865–75.

Palca, J, (1992), 'AIDS. CDC closes the case of the Florida dentist', *Science* 256: 1130–1.

Pape, J.W., Liautaud, B., Thomas., F., et al. 'Characteristics of the acquired immunodeficiency syndrome (AIDS) in Haiti' (1983), *New England Journal of Medicine* 309: 945–50.

Peeters, M., Courgnaud, V., Abela, B., Auzel, P., Pourrut, X., Bibollet-Ruche, F., Loul, S., Liegeois, F., Butel, C., Koulagna, D., Mpoudi-Ngole, E., Shaw, G. M., Hahn, B. H., and Delaporte, E. (2002), 'Risk to human health from a plethora of simian immunodeficiency viruses in primate bushmeat', *Emerging Infectious Diseases* 8: 451–7.

Peeters, M., Fransen, K., Delaporte, E., et al. (1992), 'Isolation and characterization of a new chimpanzee lentivirus (simian immunodeficiency virus isolate cpz-ant) from a wild-captured chimpanzee', *AIDS* 6: 447–51.

Peeters, M., Honore, C., Huet, T., et al. (1989), 'Isolation and partial characterization of an HIV-related virus occurring naturally in chimpanzees in Gabon, *AIDS* 3: 625–30.

Pépin, J. (2011), *The origin of AIDS*. Cambridge: Cambridge University Press.

Pépin, J., Labbé, A.-C., Mamadou-Yaya, F., et al. (2010), 'Iatrogenic transmission of human T cell lymphotropic virus type 1 and hepatitis C virus through parenteral treatment and chemoprophylaxis of sleeping sickness in colonial Equatorial Africa', *Clinical Infectious Diseases* 50: 777–784.

Pépin, J., Lavoie, M., Pybus, O. G., Pouillot, R., Foupouapouognigni, Y., Rousset, D., Labbé, A., and Njouom, R. (2010), 'Risk factors for hepatitis C virus transmission in colonial Cameroon', *Clinical Infectious Diseases* 51: 768–776.

Pincock, S. (2008), 'HIV discoverers awarded Nobel Prize for medicine', *Lancet* 372: 1373.

Piot, P., Plummer, F. A., Rey, M. A., Ngugi, E. N., Rouzioux, C., Ndinya-Achola, J. O., Veracauteren, G., D'Costa, L. J., Laga, M., Nsanze, H., et al. (1987), 'Retrospective seroepidemiology of AIDS virus infection in Nairobi populations', *Journal of Infectious Diseases* 155: 1108–12.

Piot, P., Quinn T. C., Taelman, H., et al. (1984), 'Acquired immunodeficiency syndrome in a heterosexual population in Zaire', *Lancet* ii: 65–69.

Pitchenik, A. E., Fischl, M. A., Dickinson, G. M., Becker, D. M., Fournier, A. M., et al. (1983), 'Opportunistic infections and Kaposi's sarcoma among Haitians: evidence of a new acquired immunodeficiency state', *Annals of internal medicine* 98: 277–284.

Plantier, J. C., Leoz, M., Dickerson, J. E., De Oliveira, F., Cordonnier, F., Lemée, V., Damond, F., Robertson, D. L., and Simon, F. (2009), 'A new human immunodeficiency virus derived from gorillas', *Nature Medicine* 15: 871–2.

Poulsen, A. G., Aaby, P., Jensen, H., et al. (2000), 'Risk factors for HIV-2 seropositivity among older people in Guinea-Bissau: A search for the early history of HIV-2 infection', *Scandinavian Journal of Infectious Diseases* 32: 169–75.

Rambaut, A., Robertson, D. L., Pybus, O. G., Peeters, M., and Holmes, E. C. (2001), 'Phylogeny and the origin of HIV-1', *Nature* 410, 1047–1048.

Robertson, D. L., Sharp, P. M., McCutchan, F. E., and Hahn, B. H. (1995), 'Recombination in HIV-1', *Nature* 374: 124–6.

Ronald, A. R., Ndinya-Achola, J. O., Plummer, F. A., Simonsen, J. N., Cameron, D. W., Ngugi, E. N., et al. (1988), 'A review of HIV-1 in Africa', *Bulletin of the New York Academy of Medicine* 64: 480–90.

Rudicell, R. S., Holland Jones, J., Wroblewski, E. E., Learn, G. H., Li, Y., et al. (2010), 'Impact of simian immunodeficiency virus infection on chimpanzee population dynamics', *PLoS Pathogens* 6: e1001116.

Salemi, M., Strimmer, K., Hall W. W., et al. (2001), 'Dating the common ancestor of SIVcpz and HIV-1 group M and the origin of HIV-1 subtypes using a new method to uncover clock-like molecular evolution', *FASEB Journal* 15: 276–8.

Santiago, M. L., Range, F., Keele, B. F., et al. (2005), 'Simian immunodeficiency virus infection in free-ranging sooty mangabeys (Cercocebus atys atys) from the Tai Forest, Côte d'Ivoire: Implications for the origin of epidemic human immunodeficiency virus type 2', *Journal of Virology* 79: 12515–27.

Santiago, M. L., Rodenburg, C. M., Kamenya, S., et al. (2002), 'SIVcpz in wild chimpanzees', *Science* 295: 465.

Sauter, D., Schindler, M., Specht, A., Landford, W. N., Munch, J., et al. (2009), 'Tetherin-driven adaptation of Vpu and Nef function and the evolution of pandemic and nonpandemic HIV-1 strains', *Cell Host Microbe* 6: 409–421.

Schindler, M., Munch, J., Kutsch, O., Li, H., Santiago, M. L., et al. (2006), 'Nef-mediated suppression of T cell activation was lost in a lentiviral lineage that gave rise to HIV-1', *Cell* 125: 1055–1067.

Serwadda, D., Mugerwa, R. D., Sewankambo, N. K., et al. (1985), 'Slim disease: A new disease in Uganda and its association with HTLV-III infection', *The Lancet* ii: 849–852.

Sewram, S., Singh, R., Kormuth, E., et al. (2009), 'Human TRIM5alpha expression levels and reduced susceptibility to HIV-1 infection', *Journal of Infectious Diseases* 199:1657–1663.

Sharp, P. M., Bailes, E., Stevenson, M., Emerman, M., and Hahn, B. H. (1995), 'Gene acquisition in HIV and SIV', *Philosophical Transactions of the Royal Society of London B* 349:41–7.

Sharp, P. M., Bailes, E., Gao, F., Beer, B. E., Hirsch, V. M., and Hahn, B. H. (2000), 'Origins and evolution of AIDS viruses: Estimating the time scale', *Biochemical Society Transactions* 28: 275–282.

Simon, F., Mauclère, P., Roques, P., Loussert-Ajaka, I., Müller-Trutwin, M. C., Saragosti, S., Georges-Courbot, M. C., Barré-Sinoussi, F., and Brun-Vézinet, F. (1998), 'Identification of a new human immunodeficiency virus type 1 distinct from group M and group O', *Nature Medicine* 4: 1032–7.

Smith, D. G. (1990), 'Thailand: AIDS crisis looms', *The Lancet* 335: 781–782.

Smith, T. F., Srinivasan, A., Schochetman, G., Marcus, M., and Myers, G. (1988), 'The phylogenetic history of immunodeficiency viruses', *Nature* 333: 573–5.

Souquière, S., Bibollet-Ruche, F., Robertson, D. L., Makuwa, M., Apetrei, C., Onanga, R., Kornfeld, C., Plantier, J. C., Gao, F., Abemethy, K., White, U. T., Karesh, W., Telfer, P. T., Wickings, E. J., Mauclère, P., Marx, P. A., Barré-Sinoussi, F., Hahn, B. H., Müller-Trutwin, M. C., and Simon, F. (2001), 'Wild Mandrillus sphinx are carriers of two types of lentiviruses', *Journal of Virology* 75: 7086–96.

Sousa, J. D. de, Müller, V., Lemey, P., and Vandamme, A. M. (2010), 'High GUD incidence in the early 20th century created a particularly permissive time window for the origin and initial spread of epidemic HIV strains', *PLoS One* 5: e9936.

Takehisa, J., Kraus, M. H., Ayouba, A., Bailes, E., Van Heuverswyn, F., Decker, J. M., Li, Y., Rudicell, R. S., Learn, G. H., Neel, C., et al. (2009), 'Origin and biology of simian immunodeficiency virus in wild-living western gorillas', *Journal of Virology* 83: 1635–1648.

Taubenberger, J. K., Reid, A. H., and Lourens, R. M., et al. (2005), 'Characterization of the 1918 influenza virus polymerase genes' (Letter), *Nature* 437: 889–93.

Trivers, R. (2002), 'William Donald Hamilton (1936–2000)', *Nature* 404: 828.

Vallari, A., Holzmayer, V., Harris, B., Yamaguchi, J., Ngansop, C., Makamche, F., et al. (2011), 'Confirmation of putative HIV-1 group P in Cameroon', *Journal of Virology* 85: 1403–7.

Van de Perre, P., et al. (1984), 'Acquired immunodeficiency syndrome in Rwanda', *Lancet* ii: 62–5.

Vandepitte, J., Verwilghen, R., Zachee, P. (1983), 'AIDS and cryptococcosis (Zaire, 1977)', *The Lancet* i: 925–926.

Van Heuverswyn, F., Li, Y., Neel, C., Bailes, E., Keele, B. F., Liu, W., Loul, S., Butel, C., Liegeois, F., Bienvenue, Y., Ngolle, E. M., Sharp, P. M., Shaw, G. M., Delaporte, E., Hahn, B. H., Peeters, M. (2006), 'Human immunodeficiency viruses: SIV infection in wild gorillas', *Nature* 444: 164.

Van Valen, L. (1973) 'A new evolutionary law', *Evolutionary Theory* 1: 1–30.

Vidal, N., Peeters, M., Mulanga-Kabeya, C., et al. (2000), 'Unprecedented degree of human immunodeficiency virus type 1 (HIV-1) group M genetic diversity in the Democratic Republic of Congo suggests that the HIV-1 pandemic originated in Central Africa', *Journal of Virology* 74: 10498–507.

Wain, L. V., Bailes, E., Bibollet-Ruche, F., Decker, J. M., Keele, B. F., Van Heuverswyn, F., Li, Y., Takehisa, J., Ngole, E. M., Shaw, G. M., Peeters, M., Hahn, B. H., Sharp, P. M. (2007), 'Adaptation of HIV-1 to its human host', *Molecular Biology and Evolution* 24: 1853–60.

Weiss, R. A. (2001), 'Polio vaccines exonerated', *Nature* 410: 1035–6.

Weiss, R. A. (2001), 'Natural and iatrogenic factors in human immuno-deficiency virus transmission', *Philosophical Transactions of the Royal Society London B* 356: 947–953.

Wilkins, A., Ricard, D., Todd, J., et al. (1993), 'The epidemiology of HIV infection in a rural area of Guinea-Bissau', *AIDS* 7: 1119–22.

Williams, G., Stretton, T. B., and Leonard J. C. (1960), 'Cytomegalic inclusion disease and Pneumocystis carinii infection in an adult', *The Lancet* ii: 951–955.

Wolfe, N. D., Switzer, W. M., Carr, J. K., Bhullar, V. B., Shanmugam, V., Tamoufe, U., et al. (2004), 'Naturally acquired simian retrovirus infections in central African hunters', *The Lancet* 363: 932–7.

Wolinsky, S. M., Korber, B. T., Neumann, A. U., Daniels, M., Kunstman, K. J., et al. (1996), 'Adaptive evolution of human immunodeficiency virus-type 1 during the natural course of infection', *Science* 272: 537–542.

Worobey, M., Gemmel, M., Teuwen, D. E., Haselkorn, T., Kunstman, K., Bunce, M., Muyembe, J. J., Kabongo, J. M., Kalengayi, R. M., Van Marck, E., Gilbert, M. T., Wolinsky, S. M.(2008), 'Direct evidence of extensive diversity of HIV-1 in Kinshasa by 1960', *Nature* 455: 661–4.

Worobey, M., Santiago, M. L., Keele, B. F., Ndjango, J. B., Joy, J. B., Labama, B. L., Dhed'A, B. D., Rambaut, A., Sharp, P. M., Shaw, G. M., Hahn, B. H. (2004), 'Origin of AIDS: Contaminated polio vaccine theory refuted', *Nature* 428: 820.

Worobey, M., Telfer, P., Souquière, S., Hunter, M., Coleman, C. A., Metzger, M. J., Reed, P., Makuwa, M. et al. (2010), 'Island biogeography reveals the deep history of SIV', *Science* 329 : 1487.

Yusim, K., Peeters, M., Pybus, O. G., Bhattacharya, T., Delaporte, E., Mulanga, C., Muldoon, M., Theiler, J., Korber, B. (2001), 'Using human immunodeficiency virus type 1 sequences to infer historical features of the acquired immune deficiency syndrome epidemic and human immunodeficiency virus evolution', *Philosophical Transactions of the Royal Society London B* 356: 855–66.

Zhu, T. and Ho, D. D. (1995), 'Was HIV present in 1959?' *Nature* 374: 503–4.

Zhu, T., Korber, B. T., Nahmias, A. J., Hooper, E., Sharp, P. M., and Ho, D. D. (1998), 'An African HIV-1 sequence from 1959 and implications for the origin of the epidemic', *Nature* 391: 594–597.

Zigas, V. and Gajdusek, D. C. (1959), 'Kuru: Clinical, pathological and epidemiological study of a recently discovered acute progressive degenerative disease of the central nervous system reaching "epidemic" proportions among natives of the Eastern Highlands of New Guinea', *Papua New Guinea Medical Journal* 3: 1–24.

FURTHER READING

INTRODUCTION

MMWR Weekly, 18 June 1982/31(23); 305–7.

Prusiner SB. *Science* 298: 1726–7. 2002.

R Shilts. *And the Band Played on*. London: Penguin Books. 1987.

CHAPTER 2

Apetrei C et al. The evolution of HIV and its consequences. *Infect Dis Clin N Am*. 18: 369–94. 2004.

Reeves JD and Doms RW. Human immunodeficiency virus type 2. *J Gen Virol*. 83: 1253–65. 2002.

Sharp PM et al. Cross-species transmission and recombination of 'AIDS' viruses. *Phil. Trans. R. Soc. Lond. B*. 349: 41–7. 1995.

Vidal N et al. Unprecedented degree of human immunodeficiency virus type 1 (HIV-1) group M genetic diversity in the Democratic Republic of Congo suggests that the HIV-1 pandemic originated in Central Africa. *J Virol*. 74: 10498–507. 2000.

Yusim K et al. Using human immunodeficiency virus type 1 sequences to infer historical features of the acquired immune deficiency syndrome epidemic and human immunodeficiency virus evolution. *Phil. Trans. R. Soc. Lond. B*. 356: 855–66. 2001.

CHAPTER 3

Sharp P M et al. Simian Immunodeficiency virus infection of chimpanzees. *J Virol* 79: 3891–902. 2005.

CHAPTER 4

Cohen J. In the shadow of Jane Goodall. *Science* 328: 30–5. 2010.

Goodall J and Pintea L. Securing a future of chimpanzees. *Nature* 466: 180–1. 2010.

Rouquet P et al. Wild animal mortality monitoring and human Ebola outbreaks, Gabon and Republic of Congo, 2001–2003. *Emerging Infectious Diseases* 2: 283–90. 2005.

Sharp PM and Hahn BH. Origins of HIV and the AIDS pandemic. In: *Cold Spring Harbor Perspectives in Medicine*, New York: Cold Spring Harbor Laboratory Press, 2011.

CHAPTER 5

Cohen J. Making headway under hellacious circumstances. *Science* 313: 470–3. 2006.

McCutchan FE et al. Genetic variants of HIV-1 in Thailand. *AIDS Research and Human Retroviruses* 8: 1887–95. 1992.

Robertson DL et al. Recombination in AIDS viruses. *J Mol Evol*. 40: 249–59. 1995.

Subbarao S et al. HIV Type 1 in Thailand, 1994–1995: Persistence of two subtypes with low genetic diversity. *AIDS Research and Human Retroviruses* 14: 319–27. 1998.

CHAPTER 6

Carbone M et al. Simian virus 40, poliovirus and human tumors: A review of recent developments. *Oncogene* 15: 1877–88. 1997.

Sharp PM et al. The origins of acquired immune deficiency syndrome viruses: Where and when? *Phil. Trans. R. Soc. Lond. B.* 356, 867–76. 2001.

Weiss RA. Reflections on the origin of human immunodeficiency viruses. *AIDS & Hepatitis Digest*. January, 87, 2–4. 2002.

CHAPTER 7

Iliffe J. *The African AIDS epidemic: A history*. Oxford: James Curry Ltd. 2006.

Pepin J. *The origin of AIDS*. Cambridge: Cambridge University Press. 2011.

CHAPTER 8

Ameisen J. C. et al. HIV/host interactions: lessons from the Red Queen's country. *AIDS* 16 (suppl 4): S25–31. 2002.

Malim M. H. and Emerman M. HIV-1 accessory proteins—ensuring viral survival in a hostile environment. *Cell Host & Microbe* 3: 388–98. 2008.

GLOSSARY

Accessory genes: small genes in the primate immunodeficiency virus genomes that are not necessary for virus genome replication but are dedicated to evasion of host immune cells.

Acquired immunodeficiency syndrome (AIDS): the stage of human immunodeficiency virus infection characterized by recurrent opportunistic infections.

Adult T cell leukaemia: an aggressive form of T cell malignancy caused by human T cell leukaemia virus.

Antibody: a blood protein produced in response to a foreign protein that can inactivate certain infectious agents.

Ape: large, tailless, Old World primates.

Autoimmune disease: a disease caused by immune cells or antibodies reacting with and damaging normal body structures.

Autopsy: post-mortem examination.

Bacillus anthracis: the bacterium that causes anthrax.

Base: see nucleotide.

Blood plasma: the liquid component of blood that holds red and white blood cells.

Bubonic plague: An acute infectious disease characterized by huge lymph gland swellings called bubos. Caused by the bacterium *Yersinia pestis*, it is spread from rats to humans by rat fleas.

Bushmeat: the flesh of wild animals killed in the forests of Africa, Asia, and the Americas for subsistence or commercial purposes.

Camelpox virus: a poxvirus that causes a severe disease with pock-like skin lesions in camels.

CD4 T cells: a subset of T lymphocytes that express the CD4 molecule. Also called 'helper T cells' as they help other lymphocyte subsets to generate an immune response.

Chickenpox virus: a herpesvirus—*varicella zoster* virus.

Co-evolution: linked evolution of two species, usually with mutual benefit to those species.

Cold sore: a skin lesion, usually on the face around the lips caused by *Herpes simplex* virus.

Cowpox: despite its name, this poxvirus is carried by rodents. It occasionally infects humans causing pock-like skin lesions.

Creutzfelt-Jacob disease (CJD): a neurodegenerative disease of humans caused by a prion.

Cryptococcal meningitis: inflammation of the meninges (the membranes surrounding the brain) caused by the yeast *Cryptococcus neoformans.*

Cytomegalovirus: a human herpesvirus that can cause congenital cytomegalic inclusion disease and a mononucleosis syndrome. In the immune-compromised host it may cause pneumonitis, encephalitis, colitis, hepatitis, pancreatitis, and retinitis leading to blindness.

Dementia: severe loss of global cognitive ability.

Diphtheria: a severe acute respiratory tract infection caused by *Corynebacterium diphtheria.*

DNA (deoxyribonucleic acid): a self-replicating molecule that carries the genetic code in all organisms except RNA viruses.

Ebola haemorrhagic fever: a highly lethal haemorrhagic fever caused by Ebola virus.

Ebola virus: a filovirus that causes Ebola haemorrhagic fever.

Elephantiasis: swollen leg(s) caused by the mosquito-transmitted filarial worm *Wuchereria bancroftii,* which blocks lymphatic drainage from the lower limbs.

Encephalitis: inflammation of the brain.

env: the gene that codes for retrovirus envelope proteins.

Env: a virus envelope protein.

Envelope: see viral envelope.

Epidemic: a large-scale temporary increase in a disease in a community or region.

Evolutionary tree: a branching diagram indicating the evolutionary relationship between different organisms.

Flu (influenza) virus: an orthomyxovirus that causes flu epidemics and pandemics.

Founder event: the establishment of a family of organisms from a single or few members of the species.

gag: the gene that codes for retrovirus structural proteins.

Gene: the part of a chromosome that codes for a specific protein.

Genetic fingerprinting: identification of individuals from their genetic profile.

Genome: the genetic material of an organism.

Germ cells: cells that give rise to gametes, either eggs or sperm.

Haemophilia: an X-linked inherited deficiency of blood-clotting factor VIII.

Hepatitis B virus: a DNA virus in the hepadnavirus family. A major cause of chronic liver disease.

Hepatitis C virus: a flavivirus that causes chronic liver disease.

Herpes B virus: a monkey herpesvirus that can cause fatal encephalitis in humans.

Herpesvirus: a family of DNA viruses that establish persistent infections. For example, herpes simplex virus (causes cold sores), *varicella zoster* virus (causes chickenpox and shingles), cytomegalovirus (can cause severe diarrhoea, pneumonia, encephalitis, and blindness in the immunosuppressed).

Highly active antiretroviral therapy (HAART): multi-drug therapy used to treat HIV infection.

Hominid: a member of the *Homo* genus including orangutans, gorillas, chimpanzees, bonobos, and humans.

Host restriction factors: cellular proteins that act to prevent virus entry or replication.

Human immunodeficiency viruses (HIVs): a group of retroviruses that cause AIDS. These include HIV-1 groups M, N, O, P, and HIV-2.

Human T cell leukaemia virus (HTLV)-I: a human retrovirus that causes adult T cell leukaemia.

Human T cell leukaemia virus (HTLV)-II: a human retrovirus with no known disease association.

Human T cell leukaemia virus (HTLV)-III: one of the early names given to HIV; now superseded.

Hyper-pigmentation: Darkening of an area of skin caused by increased melanin production.

Integrase: the enzyme that facilitates integration of a retroviral genome into host DNA.

Integration: the process of incorporation of a DNA sequence into another DNA chain.

Kaposi's sarcoma: an endothelial tumour caused by Kaposi sarcoma-associated herpesvirus. First described by Austro-Hungarian dermatologist, Moritz Kaposi in 1872, it characteristically presents as multiple reddish-brown patches on the skin. Most common in elderly men of Mediterranean, Eastern European, or Jewish origin. An endemic form occurs in Africa and an AIDS-associated form may accompany the immunosuppression caused by HIV infection.

Kuru: a human neurodegenerative prion disease acquired by ingestion of organs from an infected person.

Lentivirus: A subfamily of retroviruses.

Leprosy: a chronic disease of skin and peripheral nerves caused by *Mycobacterium leprae.*

Lymph gland: a tissue composed of lymphocytes and other immune cells.

Lymphadenopathy-associated virus (LAV)-1: one of the original names for HIV-1, now outdated.

Lymphadenopathy-associated virus (LAV)-2: the original name for HIV-2, now outdated.

Lymphocyte: a white blood cell that orchestrates the specific immune response.

Maculopapular rash: a red skin rash with raised spots such as that seen in measles and rubella.

Malaria: a disease caused by infection with the protozoa *Plasmodium* and spread by mosquitoes.

Matrix protein: a *gag*-coded protein that forms a matrix around the viral capsid inside the envelope of the HIV particle.

Measles virus: a morbillivirus that causes measles.

Microbe: a general term used to cover all microscopic organisms including viruses, bacteria, archaea, and other unicellular parasites.

Mitochondria: cellular organelles responsible for respiration and the generation of energy. Thought to be derived from proteobacteria.

Mitochondrial DNA: DNA found in mitochondria derived from ancient proteobacteria.

Molecular clock: a measurement of the molecular difference between two gene sequences used to estimate the evolutionary distance between them.

Most recent common ancestor: the most recent organism from which a population of organisms is derived.

Mycobacterium leprae: the bacterium that causes leprosy.

Mycobacterium tuberculosis: the bacterium that causes tuberculosis.

Myxomatosis: a severe and often fatal disease of European rabbits marked by conjunctivitis and myxomatous growths in the skin. Caused by rabbit myxoma virus.

Natural selection: as proposed by Charles Darwin, survival of the fittest leading to propagation of their inherited characteristics.

nef: the HIV accessory gene that codes for Nef.

Nef: negative factor, the viral protein coded for by *nef*.

Nucleotide: a base such as adenine, thymine, cytosine, and guanine that form the letters of the genetic code in DNA.

Oncovirus: a subfamily of retroviruses.

Opportunistic infection: an infection that takes hold because the host is immunosuppressed.

Pandemic: an epidemic spreading on more than one continent at the same time.

Pathogenic: disease-causing.

PCR: see polymerase chain reaction.

Phylogenetic tree: see evolutionary tree.

Pneumocystis jirovecii: the fungus that causes *Pneumocystis pneumonia*. Previously called *Pneumocystis carinii*

Pneumocystis pneumonia: infection of the lungs caused by the fungus *Pneumocystis jirovecii*. Common in AIDS patients.

pol: the retroviral gene that codes for viral enzymes including reverse transcriptase and integrase.

Polymerase chain reaction (PCR): a technique for amplifying DNA sequences to produce thousands or millions of identical copies.

Poppers: amyl nitrites inhaled for recreational purposes.

Poxvirus: a family of large DNA viruses including the smallpox virus.

Primate: an order of mammals comprising simians and prosimians.

Prion: a proteinaceous infectious particle. Causes the transmissible spongiform encephalopathies in humans including CJD and kuru.

Provirus: virus sequences integrated into host DNA.

Recombinant virus: a virus formed by recombination of parts of two or more virus genomes. Also called hybrid or mosaic viruses.

Restriction factors: see host restriction factors.

Retrovirus: a family of viruses that contains the HIVs.

Reverse transcriptase: the enzyme that converts the retrovirus RNA genome into DNA.

Ribonucleic acid (RNA): one of the two nucleic acids that exist in nature, the other being DNA.

Rinderpest virus: a morbillivirus that causes cattle plague, previously a fatal disease of ruminants, now eliminated.

River blindness: blindness caused by infection with the round worm *Onchocerca volvulus.*

SARS coronavirus: the virus that causes severe acute respiratory syndrome (SARS).

Schistosomiasis: a potentially fatal disease causing liver or kidney failure caused by the schistosome, a trematode fluke.

Severe acute respiratory syndrome (SARS): an emerging infection consisting of an acute respiratory illness caused by the SARS coronavirus. It is fatal in 10% of cases.

Shingles: a vesicular rash generally confined to one dermatome caused by the herpesvirus *Varicella zoster.*

SHIV: a man-made recombinant virus consisting of an SIV_{mac} genome with SIV *env* replaced by HIV-1 *env.*

Sickle cell anaemia: an inherited disorder of haemoglobin that produces sickle-shaped red blood cells. These are rapidly destroyed, leading to anaemia.

Simians: the 'higher primates' including Old World monkeys, New World monkeys, and apes.

Simian AIDS (SAIDS): an AIDS-like syndrome in rhesus monkeys caused by the simian immunodeficiency virus SIV_{mac}.

Simian foamy virus a retrovirus of the subfamily Spumavirus.

Simian immunodeficiency viruses (SIVs): retroviruses in the lentivirus subfamily that naturally infect African monkeys.

Sleeping sickness (trypanosomiasis): a fatal parasitic disease caused by a protozoa, the trypanosome, and spread by the tsetse fly.

Slim disease: a name for African AIDS first used in Uganda.

Slow virus: an old name for lentiviruses.

Spanish flu: H1N1 flu that caused a pandemic in 1918. At the time it was thought to have originated in Spain.

SV40: Simian virus 40. This virus naturally infects monkeys.

Syphilis: a chronic invasive disease caused by the spirochete *Treponema pallidum*, which is generally acquired by sexual transmission or mother to child spread.

T cell: see T lymphocyte.

Tetherin: a cellular molecule that acts as a host restriction factor.

Thrush: a superficial infection with the yeast fungus, *Candida albicans*.

T lymphocyte: a type of lymphocyte that generated the specific cell-mediated immune response.

Toxoplasmosis: A flu-like illness caused by the protozoa *Toxoplasma gondii*, carried by cats. This infection can be life threatening in the immunocompromised host.

Treponema pallidum: see syphilis.

Trim 5α (tripartite motif family of proteins 5α): a host restriction factor.

Tuberculosis (TB): a chronic infection, most commonly in the lungs, caused by *Mycobacterium tuberculosis*.

Typhoid fever: an acute infection of the gastrointestinal tract caused by the bacterium *Salmonella enteric*. Spreads via contaminated water.

Variola major: the pox virus that causes smallpox.

vif: an accessory gene found in HIV and SIV genomes.

Vif: virion infectivity factor, the protein coded by *vif*.

Viral envelope: the protein structure that surrounds the virus capsid of some viruses.

Viral fitness: the ability of a virus to compete with other strains of the same virus group.

Virus: a small infectious agent that can only replicate inside living cells.

Visna virus: a lentivirus that causes encephalitis and pneumonitis in sheep.

vpr: an accessory gene found in HIV and SIV genomes.

Vpr: viral protein R, the protein coded by *vpr*.

vpu: an accessory gene found in HIV and SIV genomes.

Vpu: viral protein U, the protein coded by *vpu*.

WHO: World Health Organization.

Yaws: a chronic skin disease caused by the spirochete *Treponema pertenue*.

Yellow fever virus: a mosquito-transmitted flavivirus that causes yellow fever, a disease characterized by jaundice.

Yersinia pestis: a flea-borne bacterial infection of rats that causes plague when it infects humans.

Zidovudine: azidothymidine (AZT), the first drug approved for the treatment of HIV infections.

Zoonosis: an infectious disease of humans caused by a microbe acquired from an animal source.

INDEX